Folens

GCSE
Health and
Social Care

DOUBLE AWARD

**Angela Fisher • Stephen Seamons
• Ian Wallace • David Webb**

About the authors

Angela Fisher is an experienced Senior Examiner and Moderator involved at all levels of Health and Social Care. She has been a consultant in the past for QCA. She was a practising teacher until very recently and has written other health and social care books.

Stephen Seamons is a Senior Examiner in Health and Social Care and an experienced Moderator. He is a clinical radiographer and practising teacher.

Ian Wallace is a Senior Examiner in Health and Social Care at all levels, Head of Health and Social Care and a practising teacher. He was also a Senior Moderator.

David Webb is a practising social worker and an experienced Examiner.

Reviewer
Glenda Hodgetts is Head of Community Studies at Portsmouth College. She has been involved with vocational writing and teaching in the field of Health and Social Care since GNVQs were first launched.

About the course

GCSE in Health and Social Care (Double Award)

In this course you will be learning about the health, social care and early years sectors and how personal development can affect our development and our health. We shall also be looking at a range of jobs in the care sector.

This course is made up of **three** units. These are:

Unit	Title	Type of Assessment
1	Health, social care and early years provision	Portfolio
2	Promoting health and well-being	Portfolio
3	Understanding personal development and relationships	Externally tested

In your student book Unit 1:Health, social care and early years provision shows you the different types of services that are available and how they are organised.

When looking at Unit 2: Promoting health and well-being you will be asked to think about the factors that can affect health and well-being and ways of promoting and supporting health improvements. You will also be asked to use methods to measure an individual's health status.

Unit 3: Understanding personal development and relationships gives you information about the different factors that can affect growth and development and about major life changes showing how people deal with them.

Working through the sections within each unit of your book will help you gain the knowledge, skills and understanding you need for the course. It will also help you prepare for your assessments.

Throughout this book there are case studies that will show you how people's needs have been met by health and social care services.

You may, as part of your course, be asked to visit health, social care and early years services, or you may have visits from specialists in the care sector. Such visits will be very useful for your course work, but you must remember that confidentiality will be very important. For example, you must change the names of the people and the care setting so that they cannot be recognised.

Your teacher may give you some worksheets to use. Some of these will help you understand the topics in your student book. They will also help you to develop the skills that you will need for your assignments.

You will collect the work for your assignments for Unit 1 and Unit 2 in a portfolio. You will have this work marked and graded by your teacher. The evidence for the portfolio will also be externally moderated. Unit 3 will be a test which is externally marked.

We hope you will enjoy using Folens GCSE in Health and Social Care and that it helps you to have a broad knowledge of the care sector. We also hope you will be successful in your GCSE in Health and Social Care (Double Award).

Contents

How to use this book

The book is divided into Units. These are shown in the contents.

Each unit has sections. These are shown in the contents.

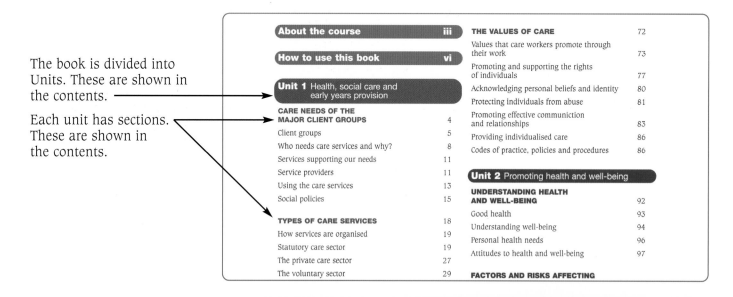

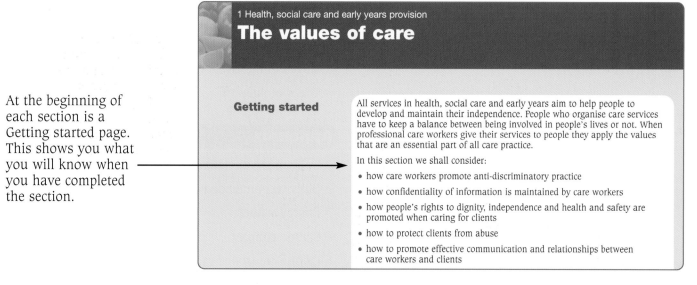

At the beginning of each section is a Getting started page. This shows you what you will know when you have completed the section.

1 Health, social care and early years provision

The values of care

Getting started

All services in health, social care and early years aim to help people to develop and maintain their independence. People who organise care services have to keep a balance between being involved in people's lives or not. When professional care workers give their services to people they apply the values that are an essential part of all care practice.

In this section we shall consider:

- how care workers promote anti-discriminatory practice
- how confidentiality of information is maintained by care workers
- how people's rights to dignity, independence and health and safety are promoted when caring for clients
- how to protect clients from abuse
- how to promote effective communication and relationships between care workers and clients

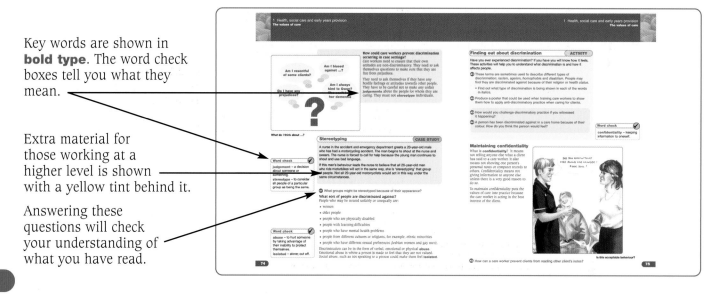

Key words are shown in **bold type**. The word check boxes tell you what they mean.

Extra material for those working at a higher level is shown with a yellow tint behind it.

Answering these questions will check your understanding of what you have read.

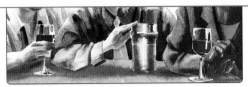

pint, and so one can contains 1.5 units of alcohol. This can be more if the drink is high strength.

Social drinking can be a pleasurable experience. It is an opportunity to get together with friends, relatives or work colleagues. We need to be careful to stay within the safe limits for drinking alcohol.

Social drinking can be pleasurable

Finding out about risks to health — ACTIVITY

A1 Make a list of the short- and long-term health risks linked to smoking.

A2 Draw up a plan to show how a person who smokes could be helped to give up.

A3 Find out the safe limits of alcohol for men and women.

A4 Draw up a plan to help a person, who is drinking too much alcohol on a regular basis, to reduce their alcoholic intake.

A5 Using the table on the next page, work out how many Calories are in a one-litre bottle of sweet white wine.

A6 What are the short- and long-term risks to health and well-being of drinking too much alcohol on a regular basis?

A7 Whole group discussion:

- Why you think people take drugs.

- Has society's view of drug-taking changed in the last five years?

Doing these activities will help you to develop knowledge, skills and understanding.

---

3 Understanding personal development and relationships
Effects of relationships on personal development

Hebbi — CASE STUDY

Hebbi has been a nurse at the same hospital for 20 years. She used to enjoy her work, but now she finds it quite hard as so much is expected of her. She never seems to have enough staff, equipment or materials. She has made many requests for more resources, but her line manager has been unable to provide them.

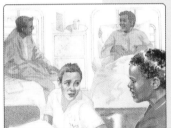

When she first started at the hospital Hebbi was happy. She liked the people she worked with, as they were able to talk about things together. Sometimes they went out as a group in the evenings. They always has a good time and seemed to laugh a lot. At work they all helped one another, particularly if someone needed help to manage their workload.

Now she is a sister she feels that she cannot be quite so friendly with the other nurses. She expects them to do a good job and will not allow standards on her ward to fall. There are one or two staff that she would, if she could choose, prefer not to work with. She knows, however, that in her professional role she needs to treat her staff equally.

Hebbi's work is important to her. She is divorced and has a mortgage to pay. Her children are at university and they

Case studies show different health and social care situations. Some show people working in health and social care. Others show clients with health and social care needs.

---

3 Understanding personal development and relationships
Effects of relationships on personal development

 ### Key learning activity — ACTIVITY

K1 From the four factors given below, write down TWO features of the relationship between Sheema and her teacher:

- power
- cooperation
- sexual
- jealousy.

K2 Describe THREE ways that Sheema's relationship with her friends could affect her development.

K3 Think about Sheema's personal development. How could her mother help her to become more independent but still protect her from harm.

Completing the key learning activities in Unit 3 will help your learning.

Friendships

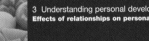

 Word check

companionship – having someone around to keep

Friendships support our need to have **companionship** and boost our self-esteem. There can be different types of friendships such as:

- close friends – people you trust and share secrets with; you are likely to

1 Health, social care and early years provision

Contents

About this unit

You will learn about:

- the range of care needs of the major client groups
- the types of services that exist to meet client group needs and how they are organised
- the ways people can obtain care services and the barriers that can prevent people from gaining access to services
- the main work roles and skills of people who provide health, social care and early years services
- the values that underpin all care work with clients.

You will understand more about the work of health, social care and early years service providers by:

- understanding how services are developed in response to social policy goals and to meet the needs of individuals
- knowing about the different services and job roles.

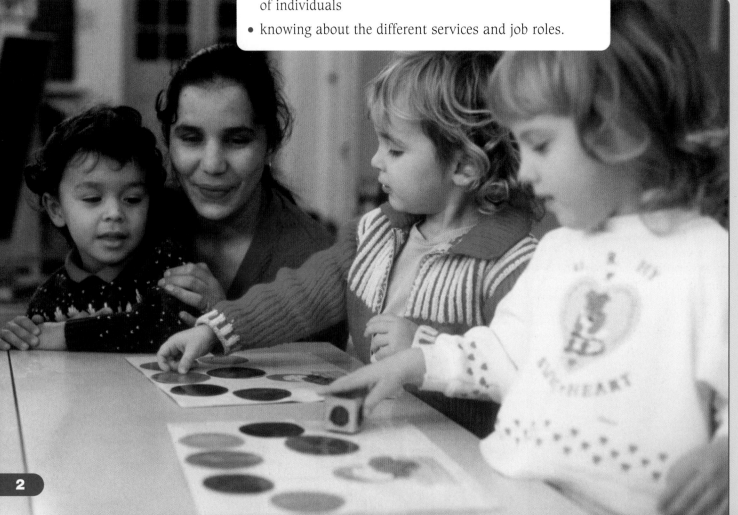

Introducing this unit

Have you ever been ill and needed the care provided by a GP or a hospital? Or perhaps when you were younger you went to nursery school. These are examples of some of the services that you will find out about in this unit. We shall be looking at the health, social care and early years services that are available in the area in which we live and at how they fit into the national picture of provision.

Have you ever found it difficult to use the care services that you need? What was it that made it hard to get the care or treatment that was needed? This unit will help you to find out what types of barriers can cause clients not to use services. It will help you to know how to overcome some of these difficulties.

Are you considering working in the health, social care and early years sector? Professional care workers who do, have been trained to carry out particular job roles. This unit will help us to find out about the day-to-day tasks that some professional care workers do and about the qualifications, qualities and skills that they need to be successful in their work.

Have you ever watched to see how a nurse or a nursery nurse cares for their clients? Professional care workers apply the value base of care within their work, so that people are treated with respect and dignity. Understanding how they do this in their every day tasks is an important part of this unit.

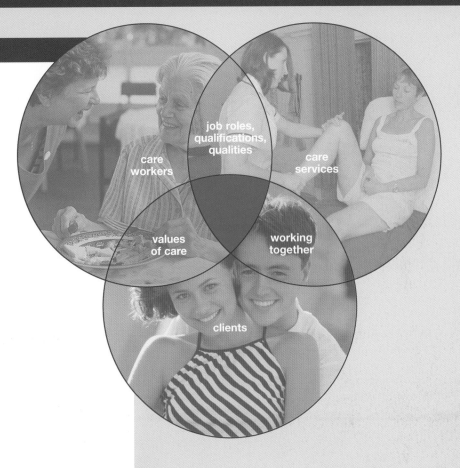

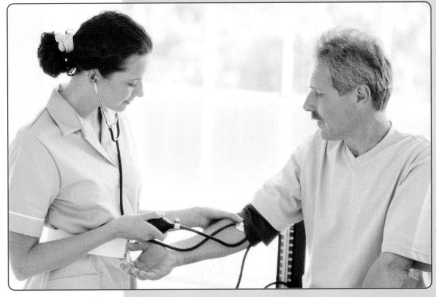

Monitoring can help prevent health problems

Care needs of the major client groups

Getting started

Who needs care services and why?

Services are provided to meet the different needs of clients. In this section you will:

- find out who the clients are

- look at the different client groups

- find out about the needs of clients in different age groups

- understand how basic health social care and early years needs are met

- understand how social policies help to influence the provision of services

- understand how health authorities and local authorities identify the needs of the people who live in their area

- find out why individuals may need to use health, social care and early years services.

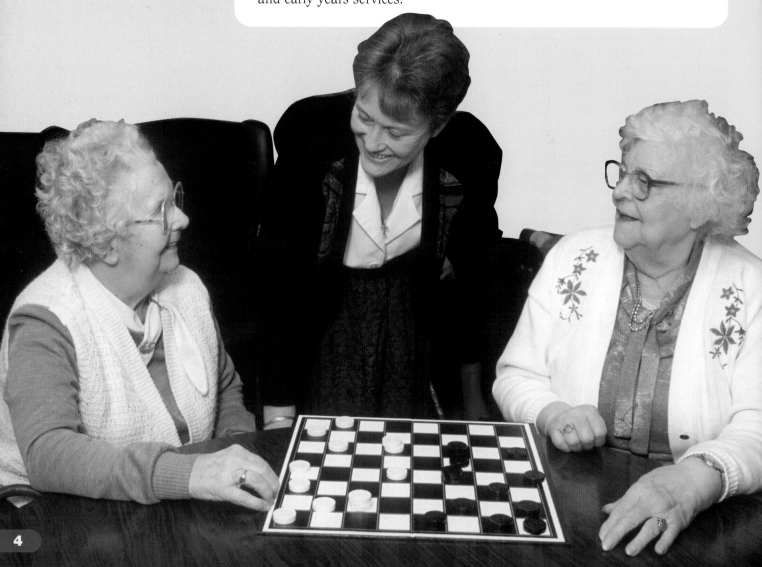

Client groups

Clients are people who have a particular need and who use services to get help. Have you ever been a client? We are all clients if we need help for our health, or for our personal needs, or if we want to use care and education services.

Clients can be can broadly be divided into:

Client group	Age range
Babies and children	0–10 years
Adolescents	11–18 years
Adults	19 and over
Older people	65 years +
Disabled people	Any age

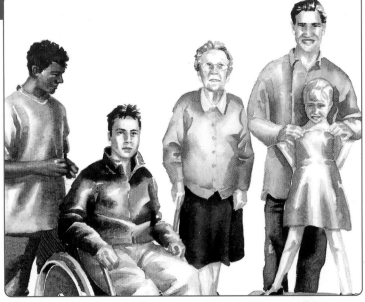

Clients are people from all age groups

Babies and children

The clients in this group go from birth up to ten years of age. Very young children are normally dependent on their parents or someone else (who is called their main carer) to make sure that they are able to use the services they need. For example, if they have to go to the GP to have a vaccination against polio.

It is important that babies and children form strong relationships with their parents or main carers. This is called **bonding**. When such relationships are formed the baby or child feels happy and secure. This security provides the basis of trust, which contributes to their emotional and social well-being.

Word check

client – a person who has a need and is helped by a trained person.

Word check

bonding – a very close link/emotional attachment.

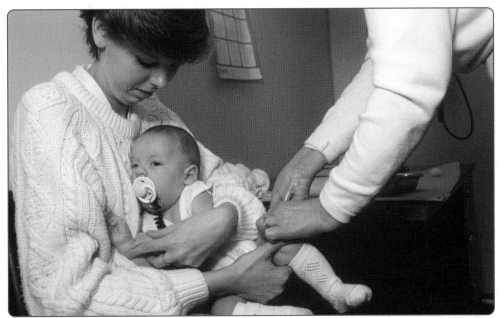

A mother protects her baby by taking it to be vaccinated at a health centre clinic

 Worksheet 9 – Who uses services?

People who provide services for children try to make sure that they are not separated from their parents or their main carer when treatment or care is needed. For example, if a baby is admitted to hospital for observation or treatment, the parents are provided with facilities, such as a room with a bed. Then they can stay to help the child feel secure and happy. The parents or carer are also encouraged to **participate** in the child's care programme so that they feel valued and part of the care process. They may be asked to feed the child or to hold a small child while it is being examined.

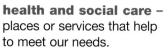

> **Word check** ✔
>
> **participate** – take part in.

Children and babies are the main users of early years services, such as day nurseries, childminders and child health services.

1 Why is it important to involve the parent or main carer when providing medical care for a baby?

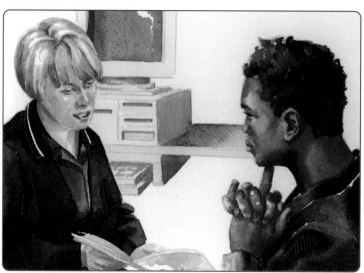

Taking advice is sometimes the sensible thing to do

Adolescents

Young people between the ages of 11 and 18 are adolescent. This stage of development, when physical growth is fast, is often known as 'puberty'. During puberty the sex hormones become active and cause physical, emotional and intellectual changes. These in turn affect an adolescent's social needs. For example, adolescents may fall in and out of love several times during this time.

Adolescents grow more independent of their parents and are able to use some services without their parents' or main carers' consent, particularly after the age of 16. For example, adolescents may decide to go to the family planning clinic for advice on contraception, without their parents' knowledge or consent.

2 Why is it important for adolescents to be able to use some health services without the consent of their parents?

Adults

People who are over the age of 18 are considered to be adult. They make their own decisions about the services they use and whether to have the treatments that are offered by **health, social care** or **early years services**.

Adults often form partnerships and set up home together. They provide one another with **mutual support**. This helps to meet their emotional and social needs as they can express their feelings and share experiences.

Adults often visit health and social care services together when they have a problem. **Service providers** must however, respect the wishes of adults if they request that personal information is not to be shared with their partner.

3 Give examples of how adults provide mutual support.

> **Word check** ✔
>
> **health and social care** – places or services that help to meet our needs.
>
> **early years services** – care and education for children up to the age of eight years.
>
> **mutual support** – two or more people sharing and helping each other.

> **Word check** ✔
>
> **service provider** – organisation that supplies help in an organised way through people trained in health, social care or early years.

Older adults

Clients who have reached a certain age are called older adults. For women this is usually at the age of 60 and for men, 65. In the future people of both sexes are likely to be referred to as older people when they are over 65. This will be the age when everyone in the United Kingdom will receive their pension from the state.

In general, people are living longer and, therefore, the age for being an older person has been changed. Older people often use health and care services more frequently than other client groups because their needs change and they become more dependent on others.

Older people may need services to help with:

- physical needs, such as medication, diet, mobility

- care and support in the home, for example, help with preparing meals, cleaning, shopping

- social support to prevent isolation and to help meet intellectual needs, for example, day care centres.

People providing services for older people aim to ensure that the individual is fully involved in planning their care. They try to **empower** the client by making sure that they are given sufficient information to make informed decisions and choices.

Older clients may want to continue living in their own homes in order to be independent. They may need support from health and care providers so that they can.

Other clients need 24-hour care and support or nursing care. They move into residential or nursing homes.

❹ Why is empowerment of older people important?

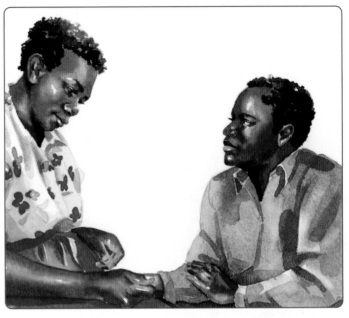

Mutual support – listening to one another is important

Word check

empower – encourage people to be independent, not to have to rely on others.

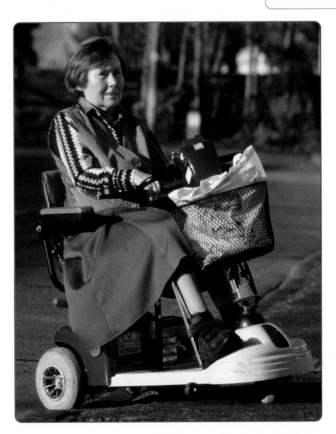

With suitable equipment older adults can often continue to live an independent life

Disabled people

People can be disabled for a number of reasons. Some examples of disablement are shown here.

Congenital condition

This is when a person is born with a disability or **impairment**. This means that part of the body is damaged and does not work properly. Deafness can be a congenital condition.

Mental disability

Someone can be born with a mental disability. Some mental disabilities occur later in life. One example that affects older people is Alzheimer's disease.

Accident

We can have an accident at any time in our lives. Someone in a motorcycle accident could lose a leg. A person could develop a sensory impairment and become blind. A swimming accident might result in paralysis.

Developmental condition

This is a disease or condition that develops after birth. It gradually becomes more severe. For example, bad eyesight often gets worse with age.

People with disabilities require a range of health and care services, for example, community care, hospital care, volunteer help.

5 How could becoming disabled affect a person's health needs?

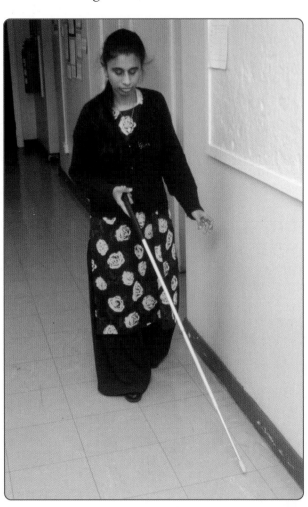

A white stick lets us know that this person is blind and may need assistance

Who needs care services and why?

We all need help at some time in our life. Some of this help is provided by care services. Think about health or social care or early years services that you have already used. Maybe you have had toothache and have visited a dentist. Maybe you have been ill and visited the GP. Perhaps he gave you a prescription to help you get better.

At any age we can have different or varied care needs. The health, social care and early years services were developed to help us as individuals.

Our needs include:

* physical needs
* intellectual needs
* emotional needs
* social needs.

6 Think about your own basic needs to keep alive. What are they?

Physical needs

It is most important that our physical needs are met. Physical needs include food, drink, warmth and shelter. To be healthy we need a balanced diet, that is a diet that contains all the nutrients that help the body to function properly. We need fluids to drink and clothing to keep us warm. Housing shelters us from the cold, from rain and from too much sun. Safety is a common need, as we need to be protected from danger.

Intellectual needs

These are needs that are met by using that part of the mind that does our thinking. We use our brains to solve problems that occur in our day-to-day lives, in our work and during leisure and recreational activities. We also use our brains to help us develop new skills and knowledge.

We all have our own interests and like different things and so as individuals we think differently. To make the best use of all our abilities we need to use our **intellect** to set ourselves goals and targets. By doing this we help to develop our **self-esteem**. When we communicate with others our intellectual needs are also being met. Taking part in activities that stimulate the brain helps us to develop and have a good **self-image**. For example, if we use our brain to solve a problem we feel a sense of achievement.

Emotional needs

How do we feel about ourselves and about others? How we feel is linked to our emotions. Sometimes we feel happy because we have achieved a goal, such as being successful in an examination or at sport. Sometimes we feel sad because a pet dies or we have to move away from our friends. Being accepted by our family, our friends and by others is very important to us. We all need to be loved and wanted and when this happens our emotional needs are being met. Being treated with respect and dignity and having privacy and independence helps us to meet our emotional needs.

7 How is our emotional state of health likely to affect others?

We should all visit the dentist regularly

Word check

intellect – the part of the brain that deals with thinking.

Word check

self-esteem – the value that you attach to yourself and your skills.

Word check

self-image – how a person sees himself or herself.

Social needs

How often do you meet up with friends to share interests and talk about the things you have done? Being able to join in activities and to communicate with other people is a way of meeting our social needs. Usually we get together with people who share the same interests. Social needs include being valued as an individual, having friends, feeling a sense of belonging and enjoying being with other people.

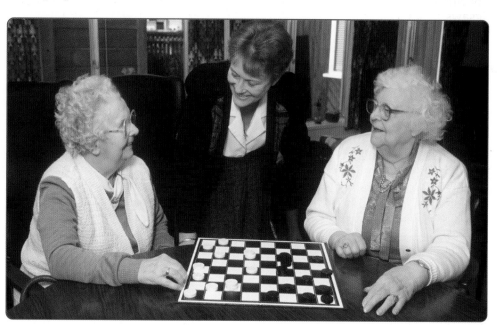

Taking part in games and other recreational activities meets our social needs

Word check ✓

culture – common values, beliefs and customs.

Cultural needs

Culture is another social need that we all have. Culture includes the values, customs and beliefs of our society. A shared culture gives a sense of community, a sense of belonging.

Maslow's pyramid of needs

Abraham Maslow suggested that our basic needs could be arranged in levels of importance. Maslow included five levels of need and arranged them in the form of a pyramid. He put the levels that he thought were most important at the base of the pyramid, supporting all the rest. Only when the basic needs have been met at level one can the other levels be met.

8 What are the basic needs of an adolescent?

LEVEL 5
Intellectual needs

LEVEL 4
Emotional needs
love, companionship, respect

LEVEL 3
Social needs
friendship, communication, mixing with others

LEVEL 2
Safety needs
protection from dangers

LEVEL 1
Physical needs
food and water, shelter and warmth

Maslow's pyramid of needs

Services supporting our needs

Different services provide for our needs in a variety of ways. For example, a nurse provides for physical needs when cleaning a wound and putting on a protective dressing.

A day nursery provides for a child's intellectual, emotional and social needs. Encouraging children to take part in activities such as finger painting, making jigsaws and playing with sand will **stimulate** them and offer a **challenge**. In this way their intellectual needs are met. Helping them feel secure by providing a happy and safe environment in the nursery where they can play with other children meets their emotional and social needs. Their physical needs can be met by providing snacks and drinks.

A day care centre for older people meets their physical needs, for example, by providing lunch for them. Their intellectual needs can be met through various activities such as bingo or community singing. Emotional and social support are met by making sure older people can talk to friends and professional care workers about their interests and problems.

People who work in care services consider clients as 'whole people'. They try to work out the clients' individual needs and then provide a service that will meet those needs.

> **Word check** ✓
>
> **stimulate** – to get the mind and body active.

> **Word check** ✓
>
> **challenge** – a problem, something that is difficult.

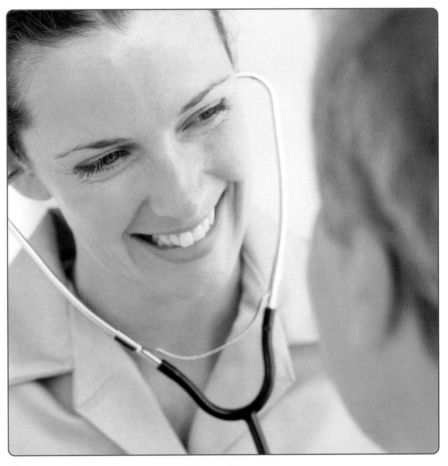

A nurse helps to meet our physical needs

Service providers

The organisations providing care are called service providers. Some service providers meet more than one of our needs while others may provide for one particular need. What health, social care or early years services have you used? You may have visited your GP or the dentist, or spent some time in hospital. Perhaps you went to a day nusery. These are all services that meet our needs whether they are health or care or early years needs.

Word check

geriatric hospital –
a hospital that specialises
in caring for older people.

What needs do services meet?

Services can broadly be divided into those that meet:

- health needs, for example, hospitals, GP surgeries, health centres
- developmental needs, for example, mother and baby clinics, **geriatric hospitals**
- social needs in day care centres or residential homes
- mental health needs, for example, psychiatric nurses who visit people in their own homes
- early years care and education needs, for example, childminders who look after children in the childminder's own home.

Majella 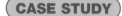 CASE STUDY

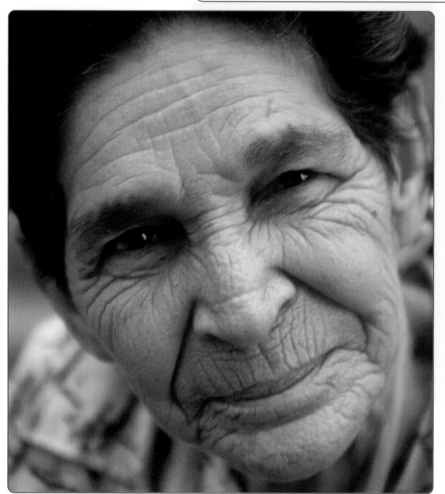

Majella is 70 years old

Majella is 70 years old. She is diabetic and also suffers from rheumatism, which makes it difficult for her to go out alone, or to do the daily tasks that are needed in her own home.

She finds it difficult to cook her meals, to take a bath, to clean the house and do the shopping.

She does not have any relatives living nearby. Her neighbour calls in each day to see if she is coping and to have a chat.

What are Majella's needs?

A1 Which life stage is Majella in?

A2 How could Majella's intellectual needs be met?

A3 Which services could help Majella cope with the daily living tasks that she is unable to do?

A4 Which basic needs does Majella's neighbour meet?

A5 Think about Maslow's pyramid of needs. Complete a similar pyramid for Majella showing how you would place her needs within the pyramid.

A6 Think of a character in a TV 'soap'. Describe their needs.

- Identify the health and social care services they would use to help meet their needs.

Using the care services

Have you used any care services? The reasons why people use services are many and varied.

They could include some of these examples:

- poor health, for example, being diabetic
- mental health needs, such as suffering from dementia
- unable to care for themselves, maybe due to lack of mobility
- health protection, for example, vaccinations against disease
- remedial treatment, perhaps to help to restore movement in a broken arm
- therapeutic need, such as occupational therapy to help mental illness
- rehabilitation, for example, counselling after a long stay in hospital then moving back into the community
- health screening, for example, to try to detect breast cancer
- developmental, early education in day nursery or with a childminder.

9 How does a day nursery help a child's development?

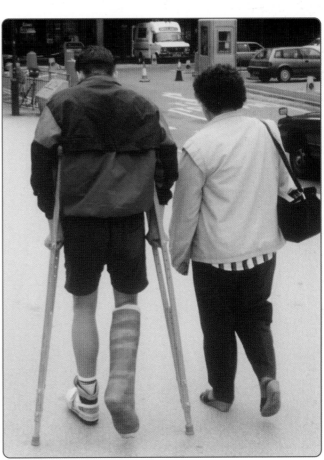

We all use health services at some time or another

Clients and the care they need ACTIVITY

To provide care we have to understand about different types of clients and their different needs. These activities should help you to do this.

A1 Draw a lifeline. Mark on the lifeline the different life stages and the age group for each stage.

A2 Make A4 size posters for each life stage. Fnd a picture to show the life stage.

- Give the main physical, intellectual, emotional and social characteristics for each life stage

- List the main needs of each client group.

A3 Draw up a table to show:

- THREE services that are used by babies and children

- why babies and children may need each service.

A4 List FOUR services that are used by adolescents.

For each service identify the different needs they would meet for the adolescent.

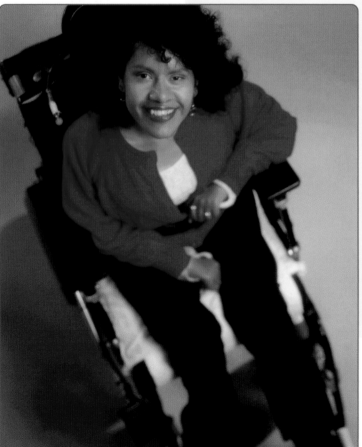

A5 Tegla is in her late thirties. She has had an accident and has to use a wheelchair as she is paralysed from the waist down. She would like to live in her own flat.

- Identify ONE physical, ONE intellectual, ONE emotional and ONE social need Tegla may have.

- For each need you list, suggest a service that could help Tegla and describe how it would achieve this.

A6 Think about your own health and care needs or those of a relative or friend.

- List THREE needs that have been met by health, social care or early years services.

- List the services that helped to meet the needs and describe how each service helped.

Tegla is confined to a wheelchair

Social policies

Have you visited the Houses of Parliament in London? This is where the UK **government** decides which health, social care and early years services are to be provided and how much money is to be spent on them. Before any decisions are taken, there are discussions between different members of the government and with other people, about the **aims** for health, social care and early years services. For example, are health services to be provided free for all those who need them? Or are people who can afford to pay, expected to pay a **contribution** for the treatment or services they receive? These discussions lead to decisions that form a **policy**. The policy is then used to help make other decisions. Often there is no 'right way' to make sure that people get the best health care or social care or early years services that they need. A policy provides broad ideas that will be the basis for making other decisions.

10 What is the purpose of having a policy?

Social policy goals

A government has a large number of targets or **goals**. Each goal focuses on a particular problem or **issue** that needs to be solved. The government forms policies about how to deal with each issue. For example, the government recently drew up a policy to 'reduce child **poverty**', to try and make sure that fewer children, in the UK, are poor. Having made this decision, the government then set goals. These are **targets** that they want to meet.

What are the government's goals?

One of the government's goals to help them to fulfil their policy to reduce child poverty, is to make sure that help is given to **lone parents**. If they cannot afford child care, lone parents may not be able to go out to work. The government is providing help through Children's Tax Credit schemes, after school clubs and by helping to pay for child care for lone parents on low pay.

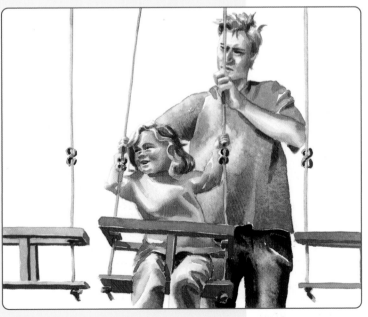

The government helps lone parents

Word check

income – the amount of money coming in to a person or to a home.

Word check

reduce – to cut down, to make smaller.

Word check

consult – talk to others, ask for people's ideas and views.

local authority – the organisation responsible for people within a local area.

health authority – the organisation responsible for the health needs of people within an area.

population – the people who live in a place or area.

located – placed or put.

debate – discussion; to talk about, to give views and opinions.

Word check

pressure group – a group of people with similar ideas who want to influence political decision-making.

media – television, radio, newspapers, web sites, etc. that pass on information.

How can a government help?

In 1998 the government introduced its 'New Deal For Lone Parents' to help unemployed lone parents get back into work. If lone parents cannot work because they cannot afford child care, their **income** may be very low. This makes it hard for them to get all the basic needs for their children. It is a 'policy goal' to encourage as many lone parents as possible to return to work, so the government is taking action to help achieve the policy they have made, by making child care more available.

What other social policies are there?

Other government social policies aim to **reduce** homelessness and drug misuse. To help achieve these aims, it has set policy goals or targets to be met within a certain time.

11 How will lone parents benefit from the government's social policy of reducing child poverty?

Implementing policies

Once a policy has been made by the government, the services that are needed to make it successful are looked at. For example, if the government has a policy to reduce drug misuse they need to make sure that there are sufficient services available to help clients.

They have to think about:

- who wants to use the services
- what type of services are needed
- which type of health care workers are needed to run the services
- where in the country are services most needed?

To answer these questions they would **consult** the people responsible for the provision of services in local areas, for example, **local authorities** and **health authorities** and others who may have opinions about the issue under consideration.

These people will look at the needs of their local **populations** and then provide the government with the information they need in order to make decisions about services.

They would also think about where the services need to be **located** and whether more people would have to be trained to run these services. There would be a lot of **debate** about how the goals could be achieved and who would be involved.

How do pressure groups affect decisions?

Some people may disagree with the ideas that are being put forward. They may form **pressure groups** to try to prevent the government from carrying out its goals. Sometimes a pressure group is formed to persuade the government to take action over a certain matter that concerns them. The **media** discuss the points made by people and put their ideas forward.

When everyone has had the chance to make their views and opinions known the government makes its decisions using all the information gathered.

Look at the diagram opposite to see how the process works.

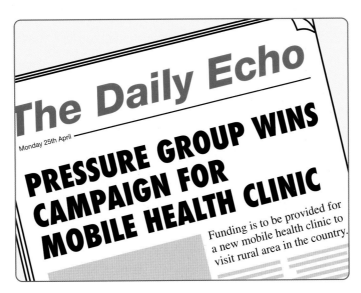

Pressure groups can help to get the services we need

12 Why are local authorities and health authorities consulted by the government when a policy is made?

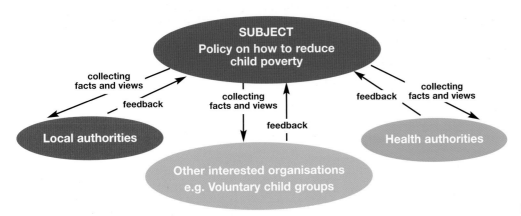

Making policy

Policies and policy goals ACTIVITY

Having policies and goals helps to shape the services we have. Use these activities to help you understand how services are developed.

A1 Draw a spider diagram to explain how a social policy is formed and the different roles of those involved in the process.

A2 Have a group discussion about the different services that would be needed to help the government reduce the misuse of drugs.

A3 Working individually, identify THREE services that would help with this policy goal. Describe how each service would contribute.

A4 Carry out some research to find out the policy goals and the actions being taken by the present government to reduce:

a) the misuse of drugs; or

b) the number of homeless people.

You could use the Internet, books or other people to help you with this task.

Types of care services

Getting started

What types of care services are provided to meet the client group needs?

In this section you will find out:

- how services are organised
- which services are in the statutory health sector
- which services are in the statutory local authority sector
- the different types of services that make up the private sector
- which services are in the voluntary sector
- how different services work together to meet the needs of different client groups
- the role of informal carers.

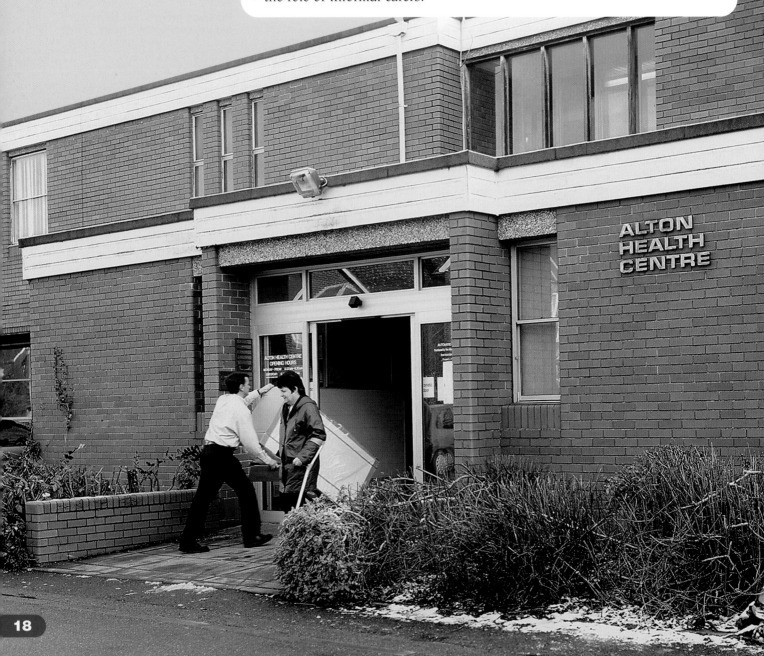

How services are organised

Health, social care and early years services are divided into three main areas or **sectors**.

Statutory care sector

The **statutory** care sector includes services provided by both the NHS (National Health Service) and the local authority services.

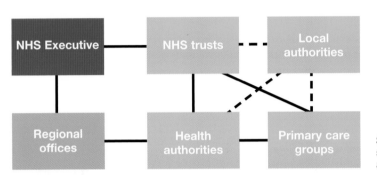

Structure of the statutory health and care services

(Broken lines indicate some links when a multi-disciplinary approach to care is used.)

Word check

sector – a part or division of something.
statutory – by law.
private – not by law, working to make a profit.
voluntary – usually working unpaid, giving services free.

Private care sector

The **private** care sector includes, for example, private hospitals, private practitioners and services provided by companies for their own employees.

Voluntary care sector

The **voluntary** care sector covers charities, local support groups and not-for-profit organisations.

The table on page 20 shows examples of services and the client groups for which they provide care.

Statutory care sector

Look at the diagram on page 21 that shows how the National Health Services, which are statutory services, are organised.

The structure of the NHS

The Department of Health is directly run by the government and has a **minister** in charge of all its work. It is responsible for health and social services. This includes the management of the NHS and social services provided by local authorities for children, for disabled people, for families who find themselves having problems, older people and other clients who may require personal support.

One of the main roles of the Department of Health is to set the policy goals for improving the nation's health. It also allocates funding and works with professional care workers and clients to develop standards of care.

Word check

minister – a person from government who is put in charge of a department or a project.

 Worksheet 1 – Finding out about services
Worksheet 2 – Where do they fit in the national framework?

Client group	Health care services	Social care services	Early years services
Babies and children	Primary health care (including maternity services, health visitors), general hospital services, mental health care, speech therapy, dentistry.	Foster care, residential care, child protection, child and family support group services.	Childminders, pre-school and nursery education, family centres, crèches, after school care, toy libraries, child guidance, parent and toddler support groups.
Adolescents	School medical services, primary health care, general hospital services, dentistry, mental health care, health promotion (smoking, sexual health, drugs, alcohol).	Foster care, residential care, youth offending services, child protection, youth work, support group services.	
Adults	Primary health care (including community provision of district and community mental health nursing), general hospital services, dentistry, mental health care, family planning clinics, health promotion (smoking, sexual health, drugs, alcohol), complementary therapies, hospices.	Housing/homelessness services, residential care, refuges, day centres, counselling support, for example, the Samaritans, and advice services, social work, support groups, service user organisations.	
Older people	Primary health care (including district and community mental health nursing), occupational therapy, complementary therapies, dentistry, chiropody/podiatry, specialist hospital services (general and mental health), nursing homes, hospices.	Sheltered/supported housing, residential care, home helps, day centres, lunch clubs, information and advice services, social work, support group services, service user organisations.	
Disabled people (additional services)	Any of the above according to individual and local needs. Additionally, specialist medical and nursing services, physiotherapy, psychology, occupational therapy, complementary therapies, specialist education and training services, for example, work-related and rehabilitative training schemes.	Any of the above according to individual and local needs. Additionally, specialist support and provision through service user organisations, direct payment personal assistance, social education, for example, life skills education and supported work schemes.	Any of the above according to individual and local needs. Separate, specialist education provision and support services are provided, in addition to integration within mainstream provision.

What else does the Department of Health do?

The work of the Department of Health can be divided into two main parts:

- to negotiate funding
- to allocate funding to the NHS authorities.

What does the NHS Executive do?

The NHS Executive is the 'stepping stone' between the Department of Health and the health authorities. It takes the policies developed by the Department of Health and puts them into **practice**. In other words, it makes sure that the services, training and **resources** needed to implement the government's policy are available.

Word check

practice – actually doing the job or work.

Word check

resources – those things that are needed, for example, materials, people or money.

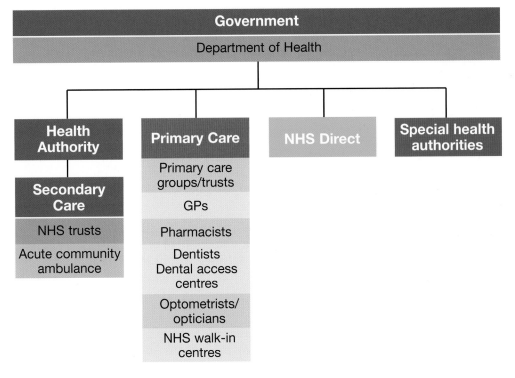

NHS services in England

What do the health authorities do?

Health authorities look after the population in their area. They receive their funding from the Department of Health and with it they buy health care for the people who need it in their area. The health authorities have to:

- **assess** the needs of people
- buy hospital and **community services** for the people in their area
- make health improvement plans (HIPs) and set targets
- **monitor** the quality of the care that is provided.

13 How is policy turned into practice?

Word check

assess – to work out or to estimate.

community services – help for local people who have health or social or early years needs but who wish to remain in their own homes.

monitor – to keep a check on, or to keep an ongoing record of something.

What are NHS trusts and what do they do?

A trust can be:

- a hospital

- an ambulance service

- a service that provides community health services (**community trust**).

Trusts receive money to pay for the services they provide directly from the health authorities and from the **primary care groups**. They agree **contracts** with primary care groups to provide health care.

14 Is there an NHS hospital in your area?

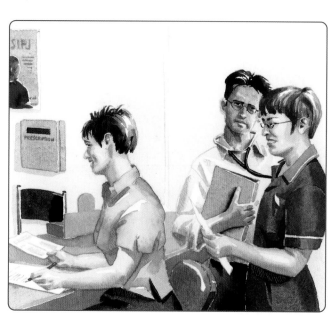

A primary health care team

What are primary care groups/trusts?

Primary health care is provided by GPs in their practices. It is called 'primary' because the GP (doctor) is usually the first person who comes into contact with a client. The primary care groups/trusts are GPs and others who have joined together to form a team. They are the people who meet clients face-to-face. They know about the needs of the clients in their area and can, therefore, plan the services that are actually needed.

In the near future primary care groups and trust hospitals are likely to join together as community trusts. They will provide both primary and community health services.

What services are available to clients?

The NHS provides a whole range of services. The chart shows some of the settings within the NHS and examples of the services they offer.

Health setting	Examples of services provided
Hospital	maternity, caring for people who are ill, surgery, x-ray, accident and emergency services, physiotherapy, pharmacy, speech therapy, occupational therapy, orthodontal clinic, opthalmic clinic, outpatient clinics, geriatric care, clinical counselling/psychology, chiropody, nutrition clinic
Dentist	treatment for teeth and gums, oral hygiene, advice
Health centre/ GP surgery	health diagnosis, physiotherapy, chiropody, health advice, counselling, maternity, family planning, giving prescriptions, monitoring health, vaccinations, immunisations
Pharmacy	making up prescriptions, advice, selling over-the-counter medicines
Community services (health)	nursing care, advice about health, psychiatric nursing, medical care, monitoring the health of children
Optician	eye testing, diagnosis of diseases of the eye, advice, providing glasses and contact lenses

Finding out about health services | ACTIVITY

These activities will help you understand who provides services and where they are available.

A1 Conduct a survey of your local area to find out about the health services that are available.

- Find out about the different client groups that use each service.

- Mark these services clearly on a map of your area. Use a key to identify each service.

- Keep the information collected about the different client groups to use in activity A2 and A3.

A2 Investigate ONE health service in detail and produce a 'Guide' to that service, that could be used to help a newcomer to the area. Include information about the services provided and their purpose. Include information about the different client groups that may use the service.

A3 From the information collected from your survey, make a list of services that would come under the heading 'primary care'.

A4 Which services provide 'secondary care'?

A5 Fiona is diabetic and has to inject insulin every day. She collects her prescription each week. Fiona also has to have regular health checks to make sure that her condition stays stable. Because she has diabetes Fiona has problems with her feet as any injuries do not heal very easily.

- Draw up a table to show all the health services Fiona would use because of her diabetes.

- For each show whether they are primary or secondary providers of health care and describe the purpose of each.

- You might like to produce the table like the one shown below to record your answers.

Draw a location map for your area

Services to help Fiona	Primary/ secondary	Client groups	How they help

A6 Carry out some research to find out about:

- NHS walk-in centres

- the work of NHS Direct

- who the clients are for each service.

T Worksheet 12 – Finding out more about clients who use services
Worksheet 13 – Putting questionnaires together and analysing results
Worksheet 18/19 – Work placement/work experience

Statutory local authority services

Local authorities are based in the area in which we live. They are responsible for the needs of people who live in their area. These are are not 'health' or 'medical' needs. The local authority has a Social Services Department that is responsible for providing services for people who have **care needs** on a **temporary** or **permanent** basis. For example, fostering services provide a short-term home for children. Adoption services arrange for a family to keep a child for life.

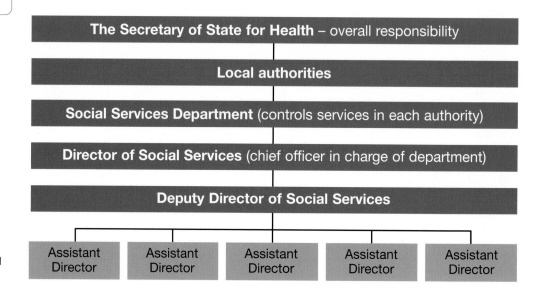

Local authority social services structure

Local authority services for children

Some services provided by the local authority for children are:

Services for children	What they do
Fostering	provide temporary homes with families
Adoption	find homes for children with families where they can stay until they become adults
Looking after children with disabilities	provide community homes, workshops, training centres
Early years	purchase places in day nurseries; register nurseries and childminders; oversee early years services in their area (Ofsted now does the registration and inspections)
Youth justice	provide youth offending teams
Child protection	care for children who are at risk, provide advice, seek care orders

Local authorities also pay for places in day nurseries for children who are **at risk** or where the family may need child care support.

15 Why are local authorities and health authorities consulted by the government when a policy is made?

Local authority services for adults

These are some of the services made available by the local authority for adults.

- **Community care**, finding and paying for places for clients in residential homes and nursing homes for people. These homes are for people who need 24-hour care and support but who may not have enough money to pay for their care.

- Providing accommodation and workshop facilities for people with physical and **learning disabilities**.

- Day centres for clients who wish to live in their own homes, but who may need to have some social **interaction** with other people.

Word check

community care – supporting people in their own homes.

Word check

learning disability – a condition that prevents the brain working fully.

Word check

interaction – being with other people and exchanging ideas.

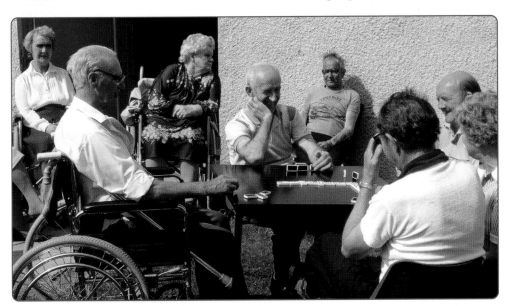

At a day centre older people can meet and chat with their friends

The local authority keeps a register of residential and nursing homes in their area.

Here are some examples of settings and services made available by the local authority for clients.

Local authority settings	Examples of services provided
Day care centre for older people	personal support, supervision, advice, chiropody, aids and adaptations, meals, leisure activities
Community care and support	advice and guidance, counselling, psychiatric support, home care services
Fostering and adoption	children's homes (temporary and permanent)
Residential care	places in residential/nursing homes
Day nurseries	purchasing places in day nurseries
Family centres	day care for children, support for adults
Resource centres for clients with disabilities	training for work, education, care, advice and guidance
Residential homes for disabled people and people with learning difficulties	personal care and support, advice and guidance

Finding out about local authority provision   ACTIVITY

Local authorities provide services for people who live in their area.

The exercises given below will help you to explore the local provision made by your local authority:

A1 On the map you used for the activity on page 23, mark FOUR services that are provided by the local authority.

   • Use a key to show each type of service.

A2 Describe the role of ONE of the services you have put on the map. This could be an early years service or a service that provides care and support for adults or older people.

   • Make sure you find out about all the services they offer, their purpose and about their client groups.

A3 Olivia is in her late sixties. She lives on her own but she is becoming very forgetful. She sometimes leaves the lights on all night and wanders around the garden in her nightdress, talking to herself. She does not eat properly and does not often wash herself.

She has no one to talk to as her family live abroad and the house next door is empty.

Produce a table to:

   • show THREE services provided by the local authority that could provide support for Olivia

   • describe how each service could help her.

Here is an example of how to produce the table.

Service to help Olivia	How the service would help

A4 Marti is four years old. Her family are having personal problems and are finding it difficult to care for Marti.

   • Find out and explain the different ways that the local social services department could provide help and support for Marti and her family.

A5 Find out what is meant by 'learning difficulties'? Find out about ONE service for people who have learning difficulties in your area and describe how it provides support.

A6 What advice would you give to a parent who has a young child with physical disabilities who wants to find out about the early years services available?

The private care sector

Private services are not provided by law. They are sometimes called **non-statutory** services. They are often set up by large companies to make a **profit**. Some offer medical care and others are involved in giving care and support, for example, counselling.

Examples of private services are:

- some hospitals
- some dentists
- alternative practitioners/therapists
- childminders
- day nurseries
- home help services.

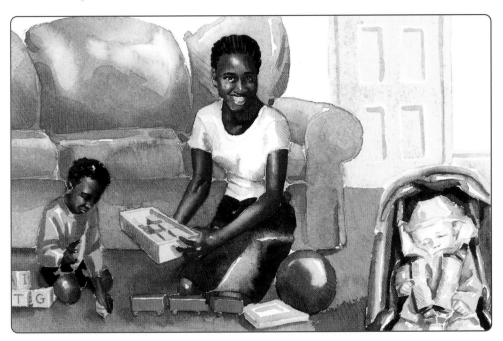

Caring for children in her own home

Private **organisations** and **practitioners** who accept private patients charge their clients for their services. Some people have **health insurance policies** to help them with the expenses for their treatment. Others pay for their treatment from their savings.

People often decide to have their medical care carried out by a private organisation, for example, a hip replacement operation, because they can choose the time and the place for it to be done. This might be important if you have a business to run or if child care is a problem.

16 How would paying to have private treatment for an operation help someone with child care problems?

How the statutory and private sectors work together

The private sector and the statutory sector often work together to meet the needs of clients. This approach is being encouraged by the government to help people get the treatment they need more quickly.

If there is a long waiting list for a particular operation or treatment, for example, a hip replacement, then a trust hospital (statutory) can make a contract with a private hospital to carry out a certain number of operations.

This means that the clients receive their operation and after-care in the private hospital but they will not pay themselves. The payment is made by the organisation that has made the contract with the private hospital.

17 How would making a contract with the private sector be beneficial to a trust hospital?

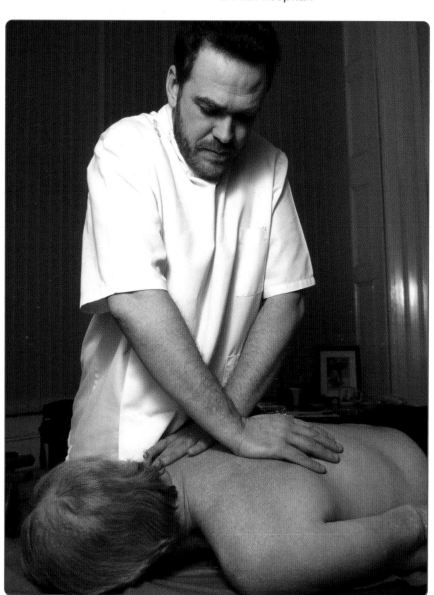

An osteopath helps to relieve pain

Have you or any of your relatives or friends ever used a service from the private sector? Sometimes people who have problems with their feet will pay to see a chiropodist privately. Someone who is suffering from back pain may arrange to visit an osteopath.

A large number of practitioners offer private services. People can make an appointment directly with a person who practices privately. They do not have to wait for their GP (General Practitioner) to make the appointment for them. Examples of practitioners who provide private treatment for clients are physiotherapists and chiropodists. **Consultants** who specialise in treating specific diseases or conditions such as heart conditions may take private patients.

Who are the private practitioners or care workers?

Practitioners who treat people privately often work in a private hospital or from their own home. Alternatively they could have their own **premises**, which have been set up with all the specialist equipment they need.

18 Why do you think some practitioners treat clients privately?

The voluntary sector

Voluntary organisations provide services or advice about health, social care and early years services, when there is a 'gap' or a need for these services, not met by other service providers. Usually voluntary sector services are free of charge, but this is not always the case. Occasionally a small charge is made for the service.

Who runs these services?

Most of the workers who give the care and advice are **volunteers**, who are not paid for the work they do. Any profit that is made by a voluntary organisation is used to make the service better or to offer a wider range of services. They are, therefore, often called **not-for-profit** organisations.

Are there any charity shops in your local area?

Next time you walk along the main street in the town where you live, keep a look out for 'charity shops'. You might find Help the Aged, Oxfam, Age Concern, Barnardo's and others. These shops sell clothes, bric-a brac, books and other items that have been donated by people who live in the area. Most of the helpers work without any pay. The money that is collected from selling the goods is used to organise services for people who have a health or care need.

When do voluntary organisations work with other sectors?

Sometimes voluntary organisations work together with the statutory service providers. An example is the provision of meals, where a social services department makes a contract with a voluntary service, such as Meals on Wheels, to supply hot meals for clients in their own homes. This is helpful for clients who are unable to cook them for themselves.

Often, when a contract is made between a statutory provider and the voluntary sector, the person who takes charge of the project for the voluntary sector is paid for their skills and expertise. This is a because a large project may require at least one full-time or part-time paid employee.

A summary of the work of the voluntary sector

- A large number of people who work in the voluntary sector give their services free of charge.

- A few people who organise major projects are paid for the work they do.

- Voluntary organisations often provide services free of charge.

- Voluntary services sometimes work with statutory care services to run particular projects. They receive some money in the form of a grant or a contract for the service they give.

- Sometimes voluntary services charge clients a small fee for their service.

> **Word check**
>
> **volunteer** – someone who works without charging for what they do.
>
> **not-for-profit** – not charging or only charging enough money to cover costs.

What is the independent sector?

You should be aware that when people talk about the 'independent sector' they are talking about both the private sector and the voluntary sector together.

Here are some examples of settings within the 'independent sector' and the services they provide:

Independent settings (private + voluntary)	Examples of services provided
Day centre for older people, for example, Help the Aged centre	meals, chiropody, personal support, aids and adaptations, leisure activities, care planning, counselling
Residential homes	24-hour care and support, chiropody
Nursing home	Medical care and support 24 hours a day
Day nurseries (private)	care and support, education
BUPA hospitals/Nuffield hospitals	surgery, medical nursing, physiotherapy, X-ray, consultations about health conditions, audiology
Community services	nursing care in client's own home, for example, MacMillan nurses
Hospice	medical care, personal care and support

Finding out about private services   ACTIVITY

Private services now work quite closely with the statutory sector. These activities will help you to understand more about how the private sector contributes to health care.

A1 Use the map you made earlier to locate TWO private services and TWO voluntary services that are in your local area. Use a key to identify each service.

A2 Carry out some research to find out about ONE of the voluntary services in detail. Make sure you find out about the services they offer, their purpose and the client groups that they support.

A3 Terry needs a hip replacement operation. He has decided to have private treatment.

- Advise Terry about the different ways that he could pay for his treatment.

- Suggest TWO private practitioners who may be able to help him to recover after he has left hospital. Explain how each practitioner would provide support and where he would go for the help.

A4 Why do you think private and voluntary organisations are often called 'the independent sector'?

Finding out about voluntary services   ACTIVITY

A1 Margo is physically disabled and uses a walking frame to help her move around her flat. Her flat is not very secure as she does not have a chain on the door. Margo is often afraid to put her heating on when it is cold in case she cannot afford to pay the bill. She sits in her coat and puts on her gloves. Sometimes Margo's brother visits, but she still gets lonely. She has a radio, but often the batteries run out and then she just sits and reads old newspapers. She cannot stand long enough to cook a hot meal. She makes do with a snack of cheese and biscuits or a sandwich each day.

- Which voluntary groups could provide help for Margo?

- How would each be able to help her?

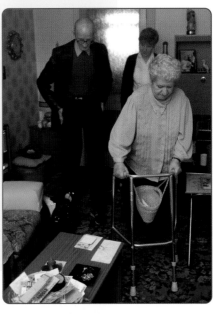

A Zimmer frame helps Margo move around her flat

Providers working together

We have already looked at three ways in which service providers work together.

The first was:

- the statutory sector and the private sector working together to provide health care, for example, the private sector doing hip replacement operations for a trust hospital.

The second example was:

- the local authority working with a voluntary organisation to supply meals for people living in their own homes, who are unable to cook for themselves.

The third way was:

- Local authority social service departments paying for places in residential homes, nursing homes and day nurseries for clients who have a health, care or education need.

The three sectors, statutory, private and voluntary are now working together more often. Those who are responsible for organising care have realised that there are major benefits from doing so. For example, benefits could be:

- quicker treatment for the client

- a wider range of services

- reduced costs by working together

- an improved service for the client.

Local care services are being 'improved' by health and social care organisations working more closely together. The 'New Modern Dependable' approach to care encourages this to happen and 'Health and Social Care Trust' organisations are being formed with the aim of encouraging **joint working**.

Word check

joint working – organisations or people from different care sectors working together for the benefit of clients.

Health Action Zones

Another development that encourages joint working are the new **Health Action Zones (HAZ)**. These have been set up to help improve the specific health needs of the people who live in the areas.

Health, social care and early years organisations work together within the 'zone' or area to improve specific needs of their population. They consider the government's 'policy goals' and try to see which are needed in their area. In one HAZ they have decided that their own local targets or goals will be to:

- reduce unwanted teenage pregnancy
- reduce domestic violence
- reduce drug, alcohol and substance abuse
- assist with transport and lifestyle issues.

How will having these goals help?

These goals will be worked on by all the service providers in the area. For example, to reduce unwanted teenage pregnancy health organisations will try to reach more teenagers to give advice on contraception. Those in education will try to raise teenage awareness of how unwanted pregnancy can be prevented. Social service departments will provide counselling services for teenagers.

By working together in this way the HAZ is more likely to achieve its goals, as there is a focus and target for all those involved.

19 What are the benefits to the clients who live in a 'Health Action Zone'?

Local communities taking local decisions to meet local needs

Thinking about a HAZ ⬤ **ACTIVITY**

Group activity

Health Action Zones have been set up by the government to help providers work together more closely and focus on health initiatives. Look at the examples on page 33. These activities will help you understand more about how they work.

A1 As a whole group, imagine you are part of a local Health Action Zone. Decide on a policy 'goal' for your area.

- When the goal has been set divide into four smaller groups as shown:

  Group 1: Health organisations
  Group 2: Local authority social services
  Group 3: Private organisations
  Group 4: Voluntary organisations

- Each group works out a plan to show what they would do to meet the goal that has been set.

- Each group presents their plan and ideas to the other groups.

Health Action Zone West Area

Priority 1 Young people/sexual health

To reduce unwanted teenage pregnancies. Our region has one of the highest teen pregnancy rates in Europe, and West HAZ has the highest in the region.

We will be working with young people to provide information about teenage pregnancy and establish new initiatives focusing on sexual health and raising self-esteem. The priority will aim to give young people a stronger voice concerning health issues.

Priority 2 Domestic violence

West HAZ will promote community safety, so that everyone feels safer in the environment in which they live. The reduction of domestic violence will be a priority, with initiatives around raising awareness, victim and offenders support and protective behaviour programmes for young adults. Also we shall be supporting running costs for CCTV in two of the town centres.

Priority 3 Drugs, alcohol and substance education

West HAZ has already employed a drug co-ordinator to work across the west area. There has been awareness training for youth workers, volunteers and members of the community and now we want to start training these people to become trainers themselves so that we have a better knowledge and understanding about what is going on and why. Soon you will see posters telling you about police/drug awareness surgeries. This is a new partnership approach so that people can feel safer about getting the right information.

Priority 4 Transport and access to services

An audit of transport provision for the west area has been commissioned to find out what is available locally. We are also looking to identify people for driver training (MIDAS). We hope that by doing all of the above this will open up opportunities for employment and local access to better services.

Priority 5 Quality and lifestyles

To work in partnership to reduce stress, tackle coronary heart disease (CHD) and improve access for those people who do not traditionally access services. To encourage men to access health services, work towards the provision of locally based accessible services by working more closely with the West PCG (Primary Care Group) and Community Health Trust. Investigate smoking cessation courses for the west area. We want to encourage greater communication across the whole of the West HAZ area.

Targets set by a Health Action Zone

Paying for health, social care and early years services

Paying for health services

Services that are made available for people must somehow be paid for. The cost of paying for the health service is rising rapidly. We often hear on the news examples of services that have to be cut or closed because of a lack of **funding**.

How are the health services funded?

They are paid for almost entirely by those who pay **tax**. This could be by paying **direct tax** in the form of income tax or **national insurance**.

Indirect tax is taken out of the money we spend when we buy goods such as fuel, alcohol and clothes.

How else is money raised?

Money is also raised by the government through charging for prescriptions and for certain services, if the client is considered to have enough income to be able to pay. Some money comes from charging private patients for using NHS services.

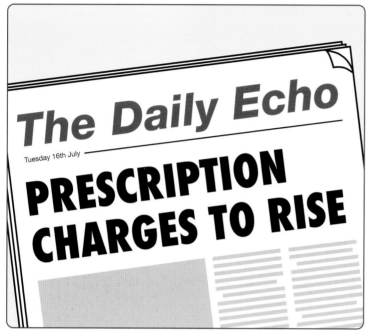

The Daily Echo

Tuesday 16th July

PRESCRIPTION CHARGES TO RISE

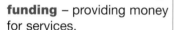

Paying for care

The NHS is the second largest expense for the government, the largest amount being spent on social services.

A recent survey showed that money for health is provided by:

- 82% from general taxation
- 12.7% from national insurance
- 3% from patient charges
- 2.3 % from sales, including selling equipment that is no longer needed.

These figures vary from year to year, but they do give a guide to the sources of money for health services. The government's attitude and its policies on health care can affect the services that are available. For example, Health Improvement Policies (HIPs) to reduce the number of unwanted teenage pregnancies, mean that more funding will be available to help achieve that goal.

It is likely, therefore, that GP practices, hospitals and educational services who make this their goal will have an increase in budget.

Money is paid directly to health authorities and to trusts, who directly manage their own budgets. When the money runs out, the services stop!

Funding varies from region to region. For example, Health Action Zones may have more money to spend on health than an area that is not in a Health Action Zone. This could mean shorter waiting lists in a HAZ.

20 How does funding affect health service provision?

Word check ✓

funding – providing money for services.

Word check ✓

tax – collection of money by government.

direct tax – money that is taken from our salary or wages before we receive it.

national insurance – money collected from our salary/wages to pay for public services.

Word check ✓

indirect tax – a tax on items that we choose to buy.

An example of how money is spent on health

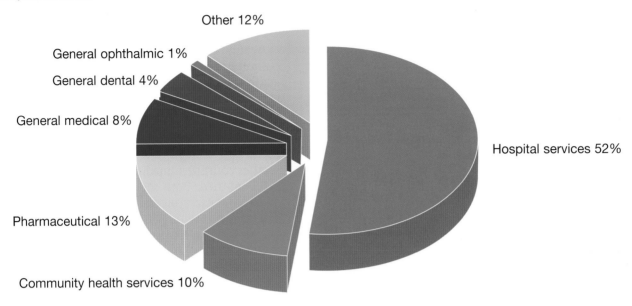

Other 12%

General ophthalmic 1%

General dental 4%

General medical 8%

Pharmaceutical 13%

Community health services 10%

Hospital services 52%

A typical balance sheet from a primary care trust

BALANCE SHEET
as at 31st March 2002

	2001/02 £000
Fixed Assets	
Tangible Assets	19 771
Current Assets	
Debtors	1996
Cash at Bank IN Hand	208
Creditors falling due within 1 year	(7031)
Total Assets less Current Liabilities	14 944
Creditors falling due in more than 1 year	(658)
Provisions for Liabilities and Charges	(344)
Total Assets Employed	13 942
Capital & Reserves	
General Fund	12 745
Revaluation Reserve	658
Donated Assets Reserve	539
Total Capital & Reserves	13 942

Income and expenditure account from a primary care trust

INCOME & EXPENDITURE ACCOUNT
For the year ended 31st March 2002

	2001/02 £000
Commissioning of Services	
Gross Operating Costs	72 272
Less: Miscellaneous Income	0
Net Operating Costs	72 272
Providing Services	
Gross Operating Costs	20 274
Less: Miscellaneous Income	(737)
Net Operating Costs	19 537
Exceptional (Gains)/Losses	0
Profit on Disposal of Fixed Assets	0
Net Operating Costs	91 809
Interest Payable	63
Net Operating Cost for the Financial Year	91 872

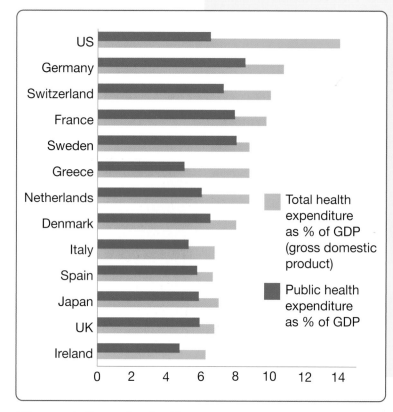

Who spends the most on health (2001/02 figures)?

How does spending on health in the UK differ from other countries?

You can see from the graph that spending on health differs quite a lot from one country to another. In mainland Europe, for example, health care is paid for by a tax on employees' wages, with an additional amount being collected from employers. If someone is not working then the state makes up their contribution.

In other countries 'medical savings accounts' are being tried. Both the USA and Singapore are using these systems. Each person pays for their health care out of savings, plus interest earned. For those who do not have a medical savings account, health care is provided by the government. This is at a very basic level and the standard of care provided is lower.

Note: Gross domestic product (GDP) is the total value of all goods and services produced by one country in a year.

Paying for local authority services

The money that social services spend comes from three different sources.

- Government grants, based on Standard Spending Assessment, which is what the government thinks the local authority should spend.

- Council Tax and local business rates. This makes up roughly a third of local authority funding.

- Money gained from charging for services.

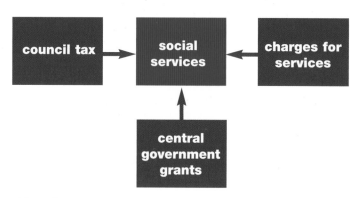

Money for social services comes from three different sources

**An example of a local
authority's spending**

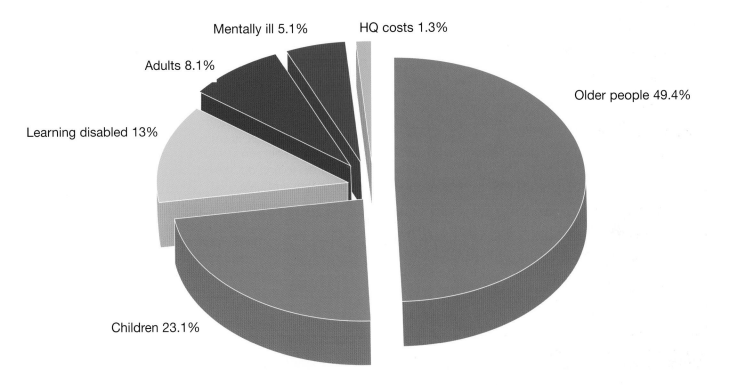

Mentally ill 5.1%

HQ costs 1.3%

Adults 8.1%

Older people 49.4%

Learning disabled 13%

Children 23.1%

Which services have to be paid for and which are free?

Some services organised by the statutory social services are provided free of charge. One example is when a social worker makes an **assessment of need**. This informs the decision about the type of help that a client may need to help them live to a reasonable standard.

For some services a charge is made. This would apply when a client requires a home care assistant to help with daily living tasks such as cleaning the house or shopping. If the client has an income over a certain amount and some savings then they would be asked to make a contribution to the cost. If the client has a very low income and few savings then the whole cost of the home help would be paid by the local authority.

How is residential and nursing home care funded?

The same principle applies when a client requires residential or nursing care. If the client has a reasonable income and savings they will be asked to contribute toward the cost of their care. If the client only has a state pension and little or no savings, the local authority will pay for most of their residential care.

Word check

assessment of need – a care worker making decisions about the health, social care or early years needs of a person.

Who will pay?

Word check

circumstances – the situation a person is in.

Word check

key worker – the main person who takes responsibility.
specialised – trained person with specific skills, to deal with particular situations.

Joan wants to move in to Hopewell Residential Home. She only has her state pension and she has no savings. The cost of her residential care will be a lot more than her state pension provides. Joan needs to move into residential care because she is no longer able to look after herself. She has mobility problems, loses her balance and does not look after her personal needs. A social worker calls to talk to Joan to find out about her **circumstances**. The social worker helps Joan to fill in a form about her financial situation. The cost of moving into the residential home will be £388 per week. Joan does not have the money to pay this weekly cost.

What is the solution?

The social worker calls a case conference. This is a meeting of all the people who are involved in caring for Joan. A **key worker** is asked to manage Joan's case. The key worker is a social worker who has **specialised** in dealing with cases like Joan's. This social worker visits Joan to find out more facts. She also talks to Joan's niece about other possible forms of care.

The social worker visits Joan to observe the tasks that she can or cannot do. This is called an 'assessment of need'. At the end of the assessment, and in discussion with others, it is decided that Joan is in need of 'level 3' care. This means that the local authority will spend money up to level 3 allowance for Joan's care in a residential home.

Joan and her niece find a suitable home for Joan. Her fee is paid by the local authority, but most of Joan's state pension is taken to contribute towards the cost of the residential care. Joan pays £140 a week out of her pension for the care. The local authority pays £248 and Joan is left with £15.55 for her personal needs each week.

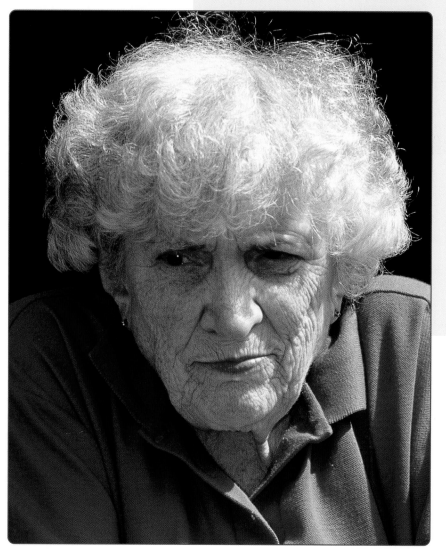

Joan needs to move into a residential home

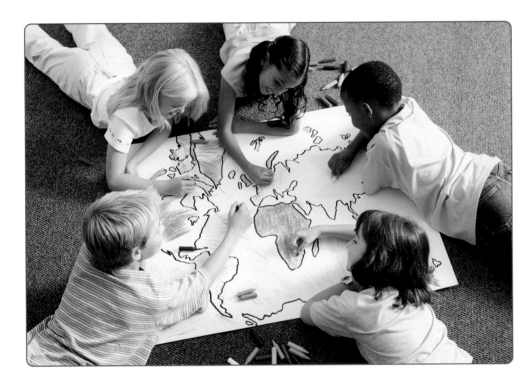

Children learn and develop
through taking part in activites

Paying for early years education

Early education charges are also linked to local authority spending. Central
government provides grants for day nurseries. Local authorities may also
provide grants and may form contracts with day nurseries, for example, for
places for children who require support.

Day nurseries make charges for children who attend. The charges vary
according to the length of time a child stays at the day nursery and the
number of children in one family that attend.

Who pays for services? ACTIVITY

Paying for services provided is not simple. The activities given below will help you
to understand who pays and where the money collected is spent.

A1 Try to find a Council Tax bill for your area. How much is spent on education
and social care services?

A2 Try to find out how much a place in a residential home would cost in your
area. You may be able to arrange a short interview with the manager to find
out more about how the service is funded.

A3 What are the charges for a prescription for different client groups? Why are
there different charges?

A4 Find out about the different charges made for attending a local day nursery?
How do the charges at a chosen care setting vary for a half day/full day
/full week? For one child/more than one child in a family?

A5 How can funding affect the provision of services at local level?

Informal carers

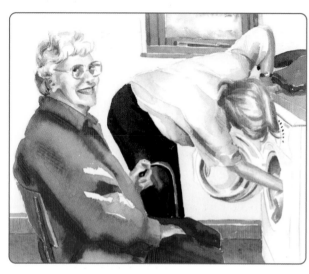

The next door neighbour is providing informal care for Mary

Who are informal carers?

Informal carers are those people who help clients without being paid to do so. They may not be qualified to care for people who are unable to look after themselves. They do so because they want to help. Often informal carers live with or near the client.

Informal carers could be:

- a relative – husband or wife, son or daughter, nephew or niece, aunt or uncle or cousin
- a friend
- a neighbour
- a volunteer friend.

What sort of jobs do informal carers do?

The jobs that informal carers do vary, depending on the type of help the person needs and the time the informal carer has. They could do the shopping, cook a meal, help with the gardening, talk to the person, help them write letters, take them for an outing, sit and look at photographs with them taking them on a 'trip down memory lane'.

Sometimes people need the help of informal carers for a short length of time, just to help them recover from an illness or an operation. Other people will require permanent help from an informal carer, particularly if they want to continue to live in their own home, but cannot do things for themselves.

21 What are the advantages of having informal carers to help with caring?

22 What are the disadvantages of having to rely on informal carers?

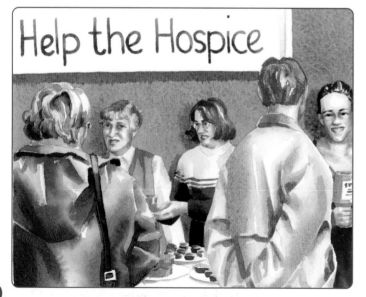

What are informal support groups?

These are groups of people who meet on a regular basis because they may have experienced similar problems or they have an interest in clients who have specific needs. Informal support groups are not provided by law (statutory) but are 'volunteers' who offer to do something without charging a fee.

This fundraising group is helping to raise money for the local hospice

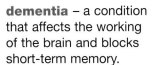

They are groups of people who join together to help give financial support or physical, social or emotional support.

For example, people may form a group to raise money for special equipment for the hospital baby unit, or a group may raise money to enable disabled children to have a holiday. People who do this are called 'fundraising groups'.

Another group of people may form a 'support group' because they want to support those people who informally care for clients on a full-time basis. They will make themselves available to look after a person who has **dementia**, for example, so that the main informal carer can have a couple of hours to themselves. Alternatively they may make themselves available to provide a 'listening ear' for a carer who may need to talk to someone about their worries and fears.

What else can informal support groups do?

Another example of a support group are people who join together to provide lunch clubs. They cook hot meals for clients, and give them the opportunity to take part in social activities.

Mutual support is provided by people who all suffer from the same type of problem, for instance, **alcohol dependency**. They will join a group, such as 'Alcoholics Anonymous'. They meet to talk about their **addiction**, and give support to one another.

Support groups can provide help for clients who have medical or care needs.

23 What is the difference between an informal support group and informal carers?

> **Word check**
>
> **dementia** – a condition that affects the working of the brain and blocks short-term memory.

> **Word check**
>
> **alcohol dependency** – needing alcohol every day; not being able to do without alcohol.
>
> **addiction** – being dependent on something, for example drugs or alcohol.

Alcoholics Anonymous

Fundraising groups

Parent and toddler group

support groups

Meals on Wheels

Scope

Relate

Lunch club

Support groups help to meet the needs of clients

Barry
CASE STUDY

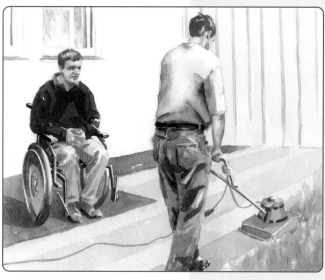

An accident changed Barry's life

Barry is 35 years old. He used to be very active and enjoyed swimming and he played badminton every week. One day while he was diving off the side of the pier at the seaside, he misjudged the distance and hit a rock. He was paralysed from the waist down as a result of his accident.

Barry spent several months in hospital. The occupational therapist talked to him about how his home could be adapted to help him live comfortably. His neighbour visited Barry while he was in hospital and told him she would cook him a meal each day once he was back home.

Barry's sister, who lives 30 miles away, told him she would visit each weekend and do his laundry and that her husband, Barry's brother-in-law, would cut the grass.

When Barry returned home a social worker called to assess his needs and to find out how he was getting on. Barry told the social worker that he felt lonely and was missing being able to meet his friends in the evenings. He was also worried about how he would get to the hospital for his monthly physiotherapy as his wheelchair could not go on the bus. He told the social worker that the GP had agreed to visit him in his own home to give him his medical checks but the physiotherapy had to be done at the hospital.

Who will help?
ACTIVITY

Informal carers provide a large amount of care. The activities based on the case study will help you explore the different roles informal carers can have.

A1 Who are the informal carers in the case study and how is each going to help Barry?

A2 Which professional care workers will help Barry to live in his own home when he returns from hospital?

A3 Describe how each professional care worker will assist Barry. What other help is Barry likely to need to enable him to live in his own home? Describe what each carer could do for him.

A4 How could the voluntary sector provide help for Barry when he is back in his own home?

A5 How has the accident changed Barry's life? How do you think he feels about being dependent on others?

A6 How could the statutory, voluntary and informal carers work together to provide the care Barry needs?

Ways of obtaining care services and barriers to access

How can people gain access to care services?

In this section you will:

- find out about the different ways of referring people to services
- think about physical and psychological barriers that can stop people from using services
- consider geographical and financial barriers that can prevent people from using services
- understand how culture and language barriers may deter people from using services
- review how resource barriers can prevent people from gaining access to the services they need
- identify the ways that people can overcome barriers.

Stairs are a physical barrier to a wheelchair-user

How people gain access to services

When you are feeling unwell and need a prescription to help fight an illness such as tonsillitis, how would you **access** your GP? You (or your parent) would probably telephone the GP surgery, and ask to make an appointment to see the GP.

Self-referral

This is known as a **self-referral**, because you have gone straight to your GP and not approached him through another professional care worker. When we want to see our GP most of us will gain access to him by taking ourselves directly to the surgery.

Professional referral

The GP however, may on some occasions want us to make an appointment with a person who has specialised in specific types of conditions or illnesses or a person who deals with injuries. He will then either telephone or write to the specialist, to make an appointment on our behalf.

This method of making an arrangement to see someone else is called a **professional referral**. Perhaps you have had such an appointment made for you if you have hurt your arm or leg and the GP thinks an x-ray is necessary. Or maybe you have had an illness and the GP has made an arrangement for you to see the specialist at the local hospital.

Third-party referral

The third way in which clients can be referred to health, social care or early years services is called **third-party referral**. This is when another person refers us to a professional because they are trying to be helpful or because we may not be in a position to get the help we need.

Leigh-Ann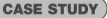

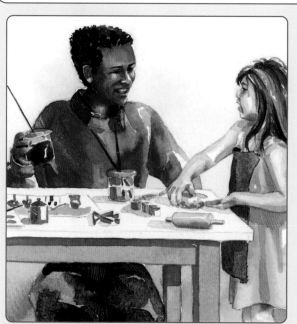

Leigh-Anne attends a day nursery three times each week. The nursery nurse becomes very worried as Leigh-Anne has bruises on her legs and on her tummy. She notices these when she takes Leigh-Anne to the toilet. The nursery nurse reports the bruising to the **named person** at the nursery who is responsible.

Two weeks later Leigh-Anne is found to have more bruises and she seems to be very sad and cries a lot. The named person at the day nursery telephones social services to report her concerns.

Leigh-Anne enjoys going to playgroup each week

Helping Leigh-Anne

ACTIVITY

A1 Why did the nursery nurse report to the 'named person'?

A2 Why do settings that provide care and education for children have a 'named person'?

A3 Produce your own short case study to include a different third-party referral.

This is a third-party referral because the day nursery's named person has telephoned the social worker. It is not a self-referral because the child or her parent has not done the referring. It is not a professional referral because a professional care worker has not referred the child. Instead another adult has done the referring and so this is a third-party referral.

What other examples of third-party referral are there?

Here are some other examples of third-party referrals.

- A teacher telephones a social worker because she has concerns about a child.

- A neighbour telephones a social worker or GP because they have concerns about a child that lives next door.

- An employer telephones a GP about a young employee who seems very depressed and the employer is afraid the employee may harm himself.

- A person telephones the emergency services for an ambulance to take an injured person to hospital.

- A neighbour telephones social services because an older person is wandering about in their garden at night and is forgetting to turn off the gas cooker.

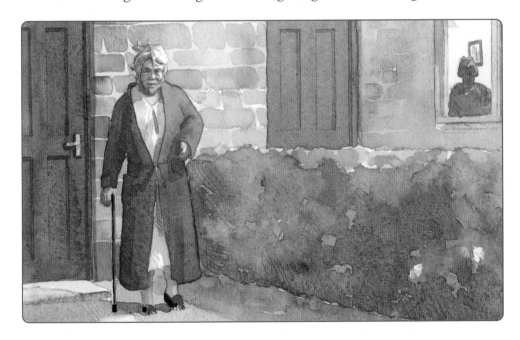

The neighbour is concerned about Norah

24 Why is it important for people to know how to access health, social care and early years services?

> ✔ **Word check**
>
> **barrier** – something that stops a person doing something.

> ✔ **Word check**
>
> **physical barrier** – some material or object that prevents a person doing what they want to do, for example, a person in a wheelchair unable to get to a GP surgery because of steps.

Barriers to services

What might prevent people from using health, social care and child care services that they need?

Sometimes people do not use the health, social care and early years services that they need. This could be for a variety of reasons but mainly because **barriers** prevent them from doing so.

Physical barriers

Imagine you are in your seventies and you suffer from rheumatism, so that you have to walk with a Zimmer frame. You want to go to the GP surgery but the only way to get to the surgery is by going up some very steep steps. You know that you cannot make it up those steps so you would probably not go to the surgery in the first place! You go without the treatment or the check up you need because of the **physical barrier** of the steps.

Some people are prevented from using health, social care and early years services because they are unable to enter or leave a building. They may not be able to use the toilet because it is upstairs or the door is not wide enough for a wheelchair to enter.

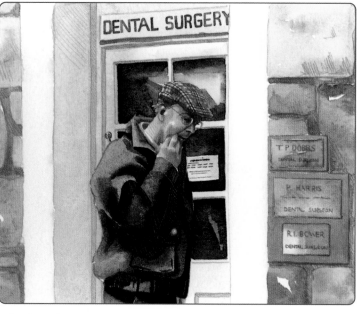

Afraid to have treatment

Psychological barriers

Psychological barriers affect the way we think. Some people are afraid of going to the dentist. They have a 'fear' of dentists. This is an example of a psychological barrier.

Some older people will not agree to going into a residential home. They think they will become dependent on others or that people will not have any respect for them because they cannot cope.

They think this is a **stigma** and will not accept the care offered even though they may know it is best for them.

Financial barriers

How often have you been prevented from doing something because it cost too much? Most of us have at some time or another. But, when people are unable to use a health, social care or early years service because of a lack of money, their health may suffer as a result. If someone lives some distance from health services, for example, the cost of travelling may be too high. If it is a private service, such as a day nursery, a family with several children may not be able to afford to make use of it. Cost can stop people from getting their prescriptions, if they have to pay for them, and so they do not get the medicine they need.

> ✔ **Word check**
>
> **psychological barrier** – fears or anxiety that prevent someone doing what they want.
>
> **stigma** – something that does not present a good image of the person.

Geographical barriers

Are you living near the health and social care services you may need? Some people live in **rural** areas and may find that getting to the services they need is difficult because they do not have a car and buses do not run at suitable times.

Older people may have difficulty getting on and off public transport, such as buses, and they may not be able to walk the distance to the service they need. They may put off going to appointments because of this and as a result their condition could get worse.

Word check

rural – a country area, not a city or built-up area.

Cultural and language barriers

In order to find out about services it is most likely that you will need to read signs, leaflets or posters. If these are written in English and this is not the language that you usually use, it may be difficult to understand fully the information that is given and so you may not know what services are available.

If a leaflet is provided by the GP or specialist to explain the treatment that is being proposed, the patient may not be able to read the leaflet or understand it. This could cause them to be come worried or frightened so psychological barriers as well as language barriers exist.

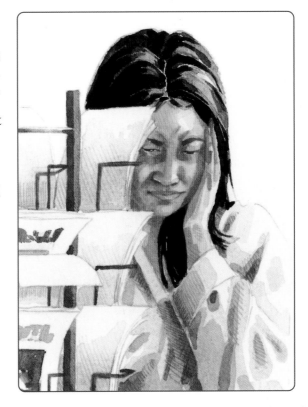

Up against a language barrier

Resource barriers

Sometimes we are not able to get the services we want because there is a shortage of staff or money to pay for the service. The lack of such resources can prevent people from gaining access to services when they really need them. Also if there is a high **demand** for a particular service then people may have to wait as there may not be sufficient money to pay for all who need the service.

Health care professionals often have to make very difficult decisions about who receives treatment. They may have one child that needs treatment that will cost a great deal of money. The same amount of money would perhaps cover 50 people who need hip replacement operations. They may not have the money for both – who should they treat?

Word check

demand – the amount of need for a service or treatment.

Summary of the barriers that can prevent people from getting the care they need.

Barrier	Examples
Physical barriers	• stairs • lack of adapted toilets • lift operating system out of reach from a wheelchair • lack of ramps • lack of lifts
Psychological barriers	• irrational fears or phobias • fear of losing independence • stigma associated with using some services • not wanting to be looked after by others • mental health problems
Financial barriers	• not wanting to lose pay by taking time off work • charges/fees • lack of money for transport • lack of money to access the service
Geographical barriers	• living in an area where facilities are limited • living in a rural area where transport is not available when the services are open • a long bus/train journey may not be realistic
Cultural and language barriers	• using English may deter some people from using services • not having professionals who are of the same sex, for example, women doctors/consultants for women • written information not in the person's own language • not knowing what is available • some treatments being considered unacceptable to certain cultures
Resource barriers	• lack of staff • lack of information about services • lack of money to fund services • high demand for a particular service

Anna and Max
CASE STUDY

Max has only been living in the UK for a few months. He and his partner, Anna, are trying to learn English but they are finding it very hard. Max is unemployed and is finding it difficult to get work, but Anna has a part-time job in the local hotel. Max and his partner have two children, Suzi who is four and Lazar who is two years old. It is difficult for the family to get transport into town, where the health, social care and early years services are. A bus leaves twice each day but the costs are high. Both Anna and Max would like Suzi to go to a day nursery, but there is not one in the village. Lazar has to go to the hospital once a week as he has cystic fibrosis and needs treatment to clear his lungs. He is waiting to have an operation to help clear his airways but the hospital has a long waiting list and staff shortages.

Coping with barriers

Gaining access to services can be difficult for some people. These activities will help you find out what can prevent people from being able to use the services they need.

A1 Anna and Max have a lot of barriers to cope with. Use the table on page 48 showing the different types of barriers that people face to help you with this task.

- Copy and complete the table by using the case study and describe how each barrier affects the family. One example has been done to show you how to do this, but you must include another physical barrier of your own from the case study.

Barriers	Examples of barriers from the case study
Physical barriers	Bus only comes twice each day so the family cannot take Suzi to a nursery
Psychological barriers	
Financial barriers	
Geographical barriers	
Cultural barriers	
Resource barriers	

A2 Think about the all the different types of barriers that can exist when clients want to use health, social care and early years services.

- Conduct a survey to find out how easy it is for clients to access TWO different health, social care or early years services.

- Record clearly the types of client that use the services, explain their needs and information about the barriers that may prevent them from using the service.

- Draw some conclusions. You can use graphs, pie charts or other methods to help you.

A3 How might clients feel if they are not able to use a service they need?

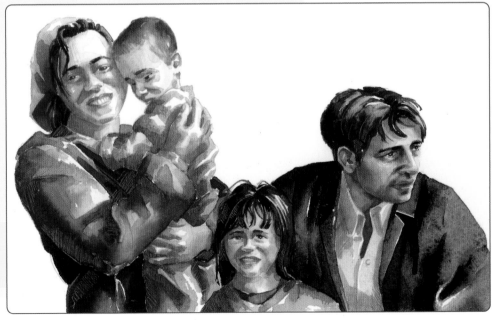

Overcoming barriers to access

Getting past the barriers and accessing health, social care and early years services is important for clients. Service providers want to make sure that they reach all those who need their services.

When new services are developed those responsible put a great deal of thought into how they can be made accessible to all. For example, someone living in a rural area may need to get to the hospital, but the buses do not run at suitable times. Maybe the person who needs to go to the hospital is in a wheelchair and cannot get on a bus. In this situation the voluntary care sector can usually help. They would organise a volunteer with transport to collect the person and to take them to the hospital.

Look at these case studies that show ways of **overcoming** barriers.

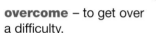

Word check

overcome – to get over a difficulty.

Cloud   CASE STUDY

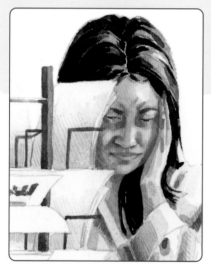

"This just does not make sense"

Cloud's usual language is not English and she cannot read the leaflet about health services.

Overcome by: having leaflets printed in other languages so that they are accessible to all.

Geoff   CASE STUDY

Geoff is in a wheelchair. He cannot use the hospital lift because the control panel is too high.

Overcome by: moving the control panel so that it can be reached at wheelchair height.

Beth   CASE STUDY

Beth is blind and cannot use the hospital lift at the hospital as she cannot use the control panel.

Overcome by: putting in a control panel that uses Braille alongside the usual type of control.

Jay CASE STUDY

Jay works shifts. The GP surgery is not open when he is off work, so he can never go for his health checks.

Overcome by: holding some surgeries at the factory where Jay works OR having early or late surgery appointments on one weekday or weekend.

Janine CASE STUDY

Janine has three children and lives on an estate, two miles from the GP surgery. She finds it very hard to get to the surgery with three children as it is a long way to walk and she cannot afford to take the bus.

Overcome by: having a mobile surgery to visit the estate twice each week so that mothers with young children and older people on the estate will not have to travel. This would also reduce the cost to the clients.

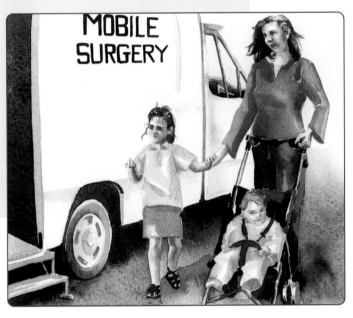

Bringing the surgery to the patients

25 Think about any problems that you or anyone you know may have had in trying to access services. How were the difficulties overcome?

Overcoming barriers ACTIVITY

It is important to find ways to get over the difficulties that prevent people using the services they need. The activities based on the case studies will help you to understand the different ways that can be used to overcome some of the barriers to accessing health and care services.

A1 For each of the case studies given provide a different way that the barrier could be overcome, describing how the suggestion would help.

A2 For each case study explain how the client might feel when faced with the barrier.

Explain how it could affect the clients' physical, intellectual, emotional and social, health and well-being.

A3 How could overcoming each barrier help to empower clients?

The main jobs in health, social care and early years services

Getting started

Those who work in health, social care and early years settings need a range of skills to perform their job roles. In this section we shall look at:

- the skills and qualities needed for care work
- direct care roles
- indirect care roles
- jobs and training for early years settings.

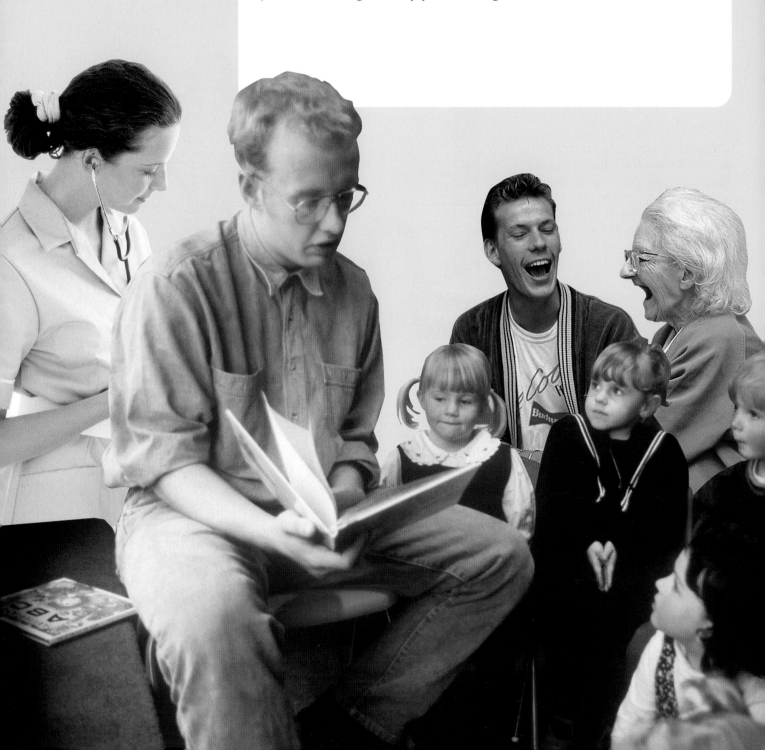

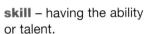

Skills for care work

Are you thinking of working in a health, social care or early years setting? Those who do, need particular **skills** and **qualities** in order to carry out their job roles successfully. Skills are developed during training and as people actually do the job.

Here are some of the main skills practitioners might need to do their jobs:

- communication skills
- scientific skills
- organising skills
- management skills
- observation skills

- leadership skills
- physical skills
- supportive skills
- skills in diplomacy
- practical skills.

A nurse's skills

How do practitioners or care workers use these skills? A nurse, for example, uses communication skills when talking to a patient or the patient's relatives. She uses them when talking to the doctor or other care workers. It is important that a nurse knows about using the right tone of voice and pace of speaking, to make it easy for the listener to follow what she says. She must also use vocabulary that can be understood by the patient.

A nurse also needs skills in management. This could involve planning and organising time, for example, to produce a duty rota to make sure there are sufficient staff on duty at any one time. Management involves making the best use of resources such as specialist equipment.

Observation skills are needed by a nurse, so that the patients' condition can be **observed** and monitored. The nurse has to make a note of any changes in the clients' condition.

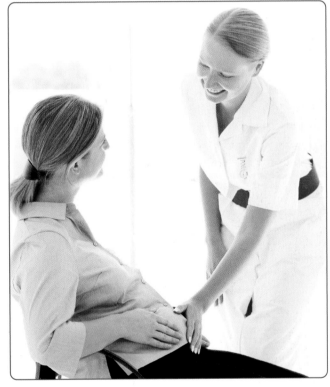

Reassuring the patient

A GP's skills

An example of leadership skills can be seen in the work of a GP (General Practitioner), leading a team of care workers such as the practice nurse, physiotherapist, health visitor and counsellor who work together in a surgery or health centre. These care workers work as a team, with the GP helping them make decisions and having overall responsibility for any decisions that are made.

A GP also requires scientific skills. He has to understand about the different types of **medication** and their effects on patients. This is so that clients are given the best treatment for their condition or illness.

 Worksheet 5 – Finding out about jobs in a medical centre
Worksheet 7 – How do you become a care worker?

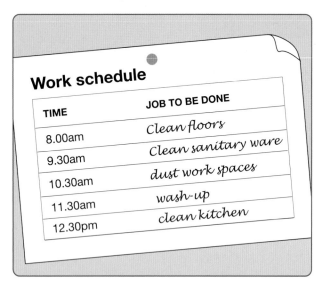

Work schedule

TIME	JOB TO BE DONE
8.00am	Clean floors
9.30am	Clean sanitary ware
10.30am	dust work spaces
11.30am	wash-up
12.30pm	clean kitchen

It is important to work out the best order to do things

Word check ✓

common – shared by two or more people

A care assistant's skills

Care assistants need physical skills, to be able to clean and prepare clients' rooms. They also need skills of communication so that they can talk to clients in order to meet their social and emotional needs. They also need organisational skills, so they can plan their work and make best use of their time.

What skills are common to all care workers?

Some skills are **common** to all care workers. One example is skills in 'diplomacy'. This is important when giving people upsetting news or when a client is upset, angry or afraid. The care worker must be careful to use words that will not upset the person more. To give another example, the care worker should not say anything that makes it look as though they are supporting the view of one client against another, or one care worker against another.

26 Which other skills might be common to all care workers?

What is the difference between a skill and a quality?

A quality is something that is part of us, a part that makes us what we are. For example, someone may say, 'Oh, she is always very kind'. Being kind is a characteristic or quality that a person has. What qualities do you have? Are you honest, reliable, hard-working, truthful, calm? Do you have an ability to get on well with others or to cope with difficult situations? These are all personal qualities that make us different from other people. Some of these are needed for working in health, social care and early years services. We may not have all of these qualities but we usually have some of them.

Another quality that is always helpful is a sense of humour. Not all of us possess a sense of humour, but being able to see the funny side of something can often help a situation.

27 How can qualities contribute to the job role of a care worker?

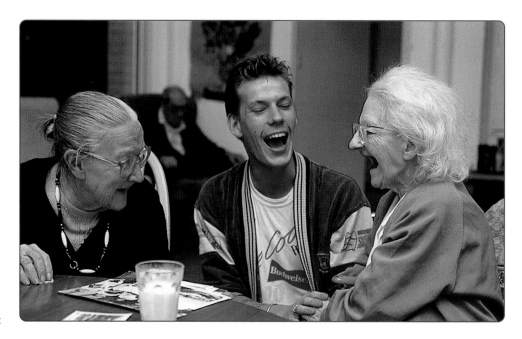

A sense of humour is important

Jobs in health and social care

Jobs can be divided into:

- **direct care roles** – these are jobs where the practitioner is in personal contact with the client. Examples are: nurse, doctor, social worker and care assistant. There are, of course, many other job roles.

- **indirect care roles** – these are jobs where the person gives support to those who are personally or directly caring for clients. Examples of these jobs are receptionist, porter and cleaner.

Both direct and indirect care roles are important as the client can only receive the best care when both are working together to **promote** the interest of the client.

Let us look at the job roles of some of the practitioners who work in health.

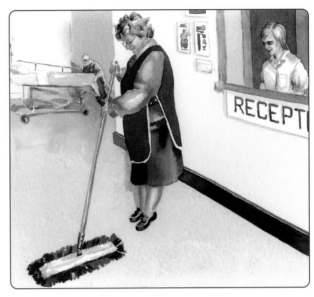

Indirect care – people who provide support in care settings

The work of a registered nurse

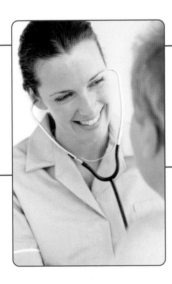

Qualifications

- degree in nursing or three-year nursing course. To get on the training course five GCSEs are required

Skills

- communication skills
- practical skills
- skills in diplomacy
- observation skills
- scientific skills

Qualities

- calmness
- reliability
- sense of humour
- patience

Working at

- hospital
- health centre
- clinic
- nursing home

Word check

direct care role – a job with the responsibility for the care of patients or clients.

Word check

indirect care role – helping to care for a patient or client by providing support.

Word check

promote – to put forward.

What does a registered nurse do?

- assists with clients' medical treatment
- assesses patients' health and care needs
- writes reports and care plans
- talks to clients and relatives
- looks after the general care of clients
- monitors clients' health
- accompanies doctors on their rounds of the ward.

Gemma's day as a nurse at Hopewell Hospital

CASE STUDY

I start work at the hospital at 8:00am and work through until 4:00pm. I get an hour for lunch and two coffee breaks. When I come on duty I have a meeting with the sister and the other nurses on the ward to find out what has happened to the patients during the night. We discuss the patients' care plans and the sister will recommend changes to them, if necessary.

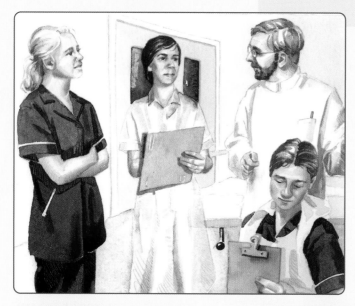

It is important that everyone who works on the ward knows about each patient's needs

I greet all the patients on the ward and ask them how they are. I usually tell them what the weather is like. The patients will have had their breakfast so my first job is to make sure all the breakfast things are removed and then to help the patients get washed. Some are able to go to the bathroom by themselves, but others need help with washing.

Some patients need bedpans and I have to help them to sit comfortably on these and empty them when the client has finished. I work with other nurses to do this as we are not allowed to lift patients on our own.

I then have to make sure that the beds are made properly and that each patient is comfortable.

The patients are left to sleep or to read or watch TV while I check their records and make sure these are in order for the doctors' rounds. The doctors do the rounds of the wards between 9:30am and 11:00am. I go around with them and answer their questions about the medication the patient has received and tell them about any changes in the patient's condition. The doctor talks to the person and asks them how they feel. The doctor then decides whether there is to be any change in medication or treatment for that person.

At around 11:00am the tea and coffee trolley arrives and I help to make sure that everyone gets the drink they want.

Some patients need a dressing changed or to be prepared for physiotherapy or surgery.

Lunch arrives around 12:30pm. I make sure that patients who have to remain in bed are in a comfortable position to eat their lunch. Some may need feeding and I help to do this.

Throughout the day I am talking to all the people in the ward and trying to brighten up their day. Some are worried about their condition or about the treatment they are to have. I try to support them by reassuring them and explaining exactly what is going to happen. I find people are not so afraid if they know the facts.

After lunch we monitor the patients' health by taking their temperatures and pulse. We record these on charts. Some patients need medication. I accompany the sister who is giving it out to check that the correct medication, in the right amount is being given to the right person.

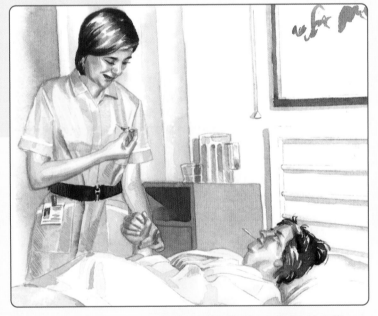

Monitoring patients' health is an important part of the job

Visiting time starts at 2:00pm. At this time I make sure that all the records are up to date. I also chat with patients who do not have any visitors. Sometimes I have to change more dressings or help patients who are feeling very unwell.

Before going off duty I have a meeting with the staff who are coming on duty so that we can exchange information about the patients' health and the treatment and medication they have received.

Finding out about Gemma's work ACTIVITY

Gemma works hard in her job and likes what she does. The activities below will help you to look carefully at the day-to-day tasks she does.

A1 List FIVE skills used by Gemma in her job role.

A2 List FIVE qualities that would help Gemma in her job.

A3 When during her day would Gemma have to use diplomacy skills?

A4 How does Gemma form good relationships with the patients?

A5 Imagine you are a patient on Gemma's ward. What are your needs? How could Gemma meet your needs?

Word check

care setting – a place where people are cared for or looked after.

Word check

oral hygienist – a person whose role is to attend to the hygiene of clients' teeth, gums and mouth.

Direct care roles in health settings

As you have seen already in this section there is a wide range of job roles within the health sector. Care workers carry out their jobs in different **care settings** such as hospitals, clinics, GP surgeries, health centres, dental surgeries and opticians. Within each setting some job roles involve direct caring for clients and others are support or indirect care roles. Let us look at some 'snapshots' of different direct care roles in health settings.

Mr Danby, dentist CASE STUDY

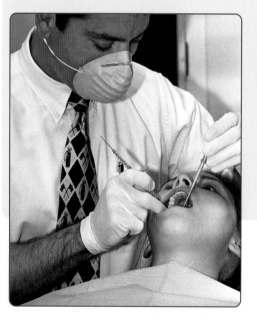

Dentists needs to be able to communicate with their patients

I work in a dental practice with three other dentists and an **oral hygienist**. We try to take care of people's teeth. We sometimes have to fill a tooth if a hole (cavity) is causing toothache. Occasionally we have to remove teeth if they are broken off or beyond repair. We try to give advice to people about how to look after their teeth so that they will not need fillings or to have their teeth removed. I have a degree in dentistry and post-graduate training.

28 What skills and qualities would be required by a dentist?

29 How do people become dentists?

Mrs Wallace, optician

My shop is in the high street. Most people think that my main job is to help them choose their glasses frames, but my assistants do that. I test the client's eyesight and as I am doing this I also check for eye diseases and conditions such as squints and **double vision**. I have to know how to use the equipment that helps me to make a **diagnosis**. If I think there are really major problems I refer the client to a specialist. I have to make sure that the client has the correct strength of lens – if the prescription is not accurate damage could be caused to the eye. I have to be very precise in my work and pay attention to detail. My training was quite long; I have a degree in optometry and other **ophthalmic** qualifications. I have my own shop, but opticians work in hospitals, clinics or **laboratories**.

Word check	

double vision – seeing two of everything.
diagnosis – identifying what the problem is.
ophthalmic – relating to the eye.
laboratory – building or room equipped for scientific research or experiments.

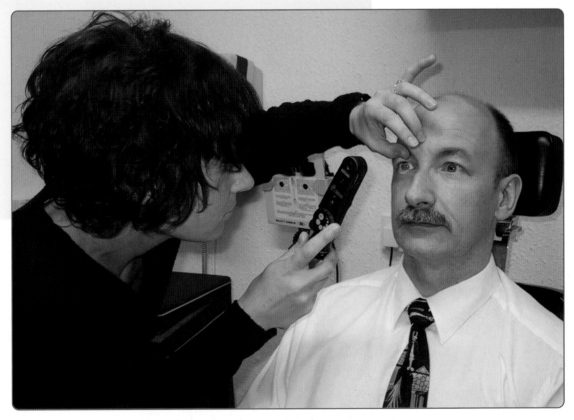

Improving people's sight

30 How is the work of an optician different from that of a dentist?

31 What skills are common to both opticians and dentists?

Word check

massage – using the hands to rub, knead and manipulate parts of the client's body.

Christine Baker, physiotherapist ⬤ CASE STUDY

I work at the local hospital where I design programmes of exercise for patients who have broken bones or muscle injuries to help strengthen the injured part. Sometimes I use heat and **massage** to aid the treatment.

I have to keep very careful records of the exercises each patient does and of the effects these seem to be having on the injured part. I must make sure that the patient understands how to do the exercises correctly, so communication skills and getting on with clients is a very important aspect of my work. I have a degree in physiotherapy and also a qualification in remedial gymnastics. My friend who works in the same hospital does not have a degree. He became a physiotherapist's aide and did a lot of on-the-job training. He then took a three-year course in physiotherapy and gained his qualification in that way.

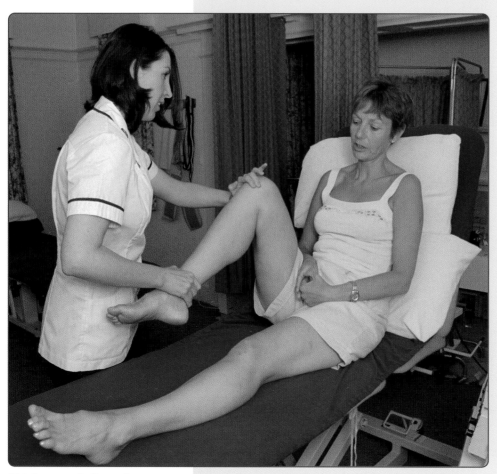

Helping people through exercises and massage

Getting to know about jobs (ACTIVITY)

Different skills and qualities are needed for different jobs. In these activities we shall find out what tasks people do and the skills and qualities needed to do them.

A1 Research: finding out about jobs

- Copy and complete the table to show the skills and qualities needed, and the main tasks carried out by care workers. You will need to make the table much larger.

Job role	Skills	Qualities	Main tasks
GP			
District nurse			
Health visitor			
Midwife			
Physiotherapist			
Radiologist			

A2 Find out about the day-to-day tasks of one care worker in the health sector. If possible collect your evidence through conducting an interview with the person doing the job. If you use this method to collect evidence you will need to plan the questions you ask to make sure that you get all the information required.

A3 How different is the job of a nurse in a surgical ward from that of a nurse on a children's ward? Compare the skills each would use.

Indirect care roles in health settings

Medical receptionist

- answers telephone
- makes appointments for clients
- gives directions to clients
- answers questions

Cleaner

- brushes/mops floor
- dusts surfaces
- talks to clients
- cleans basins, baths and toilets

Porter

- moves clients from ward to treatment rooms
- moves equipment
- talks to clients
- helps to set up equipment

Who are indirect care workers?

People working as indirect care workers are very important. Without them the practitioners would not be able to do their jobs successfully. The receptionist, for example, may be the first person to greet a client and may influence the first impression a client forms of the care setting and the people who work there. The receptionist needs good communication skills. Greeting people, making them feel welcome and directing them to the care worker they need are important aspects of their role.

Aubrey, porter
CASE STUDY

I enjoy my work as each day is different. I sign in at 7:00am and finish at a quarter to four. I have a contact radio and when I am needed I get a call on my radio. Sometimes I have to collect a parcel or equipment. At other times I will be asked to take a patient down in the lift to the x-ray department. I try to talk to the patient if they are well enough as this cheers them up and stops them worrying about what is going to happen next. I meet some interesting people in my work.

32 What skills is Aubrey using in his job as a porter?

Alison, supervisory cleaner at Hopewell Hospital
CASE STUDY

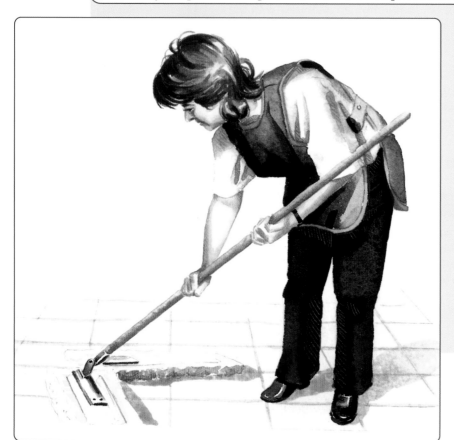

I work from 8:00am until midday.

I have to clean three wards and the washbasins and bathrooms. I have to make sure that I don't make too much dust as this could harm the patient, so I damp mop around the beds. I sometimes talk to the patients if they are not too ill. I don't talk to them too much because I don't want to make them tired but they do like me to say 'hello', especially the older ones. My work is only part-time but I do like it. I like to see the wards looking clean when I've finished.

I also have to see that the other people who are employed as cleaners complete their jobs to a high standard. I work out job schedules and draw up a duty rota for my team.

33 What are the differences between direct and indirect care roles?

A cleaner's role is an important part of the hospital's hygiene routines

Care workers in social care roles

Social care workers provide support for people. Their clients may have health problems but it is not part of the social care worker's job role to be involved with the treatment of their medical condition or illness. Their work may result from a health problem or the client may only have social care related needs.

Job roles in social care

What jobs are there in social care? The table shows you some of the main roles and the main tasks carried out by the practitioner and the skills needed.

Job	Main tasks	Skills required
Care assistant in a day centre	• welcoming clients • helping them order their lunch • talking to clients • providing activities for clients	• communication • practical problem solving • organising • planning • listening • **assertiveness**
Social worker	• listening to clients • providing advice/information • putting clients in touch with other agencies • assessing clients' needs • organising support services for clients	• communication • diplomacy • listening • problem solving • observation • management • leadership
Domiciliary care assistant (home care)	• shopping for clients • cleaning and tidying rooms • helping to sort clothes • ironing • writing letters • talking to clients	• mathematical • practical • organising • diplomacy • communication • problem solving • **flexibility**
Residential care assistant	• helping to get clients up in the morning • helping with feeding • talking to clients • taking clients for walks • preparing drinks and light snacks for clients • observation	• practical • listening • interpersonal • communication • diplomacy • supportive • assertiveness

Word check ✓

assertiveness – being firm and confident.

Word check ✓

flexibility – able to adapt; not having to keep to the same routine.

How do people become social workers?

Anyone wanting to be a social worker cannot start training until they are 21 years old. Before that age, those who want to train are encouraged to take jobs where they can help people so that they can gain experience of working with others. When training is complete the social worker will have a 'Diploma in Social Work'.

34 Why do you think people who want to become social workers should have some 'life experience' before starting their training?

Worksheet 6 – Finding out about jobs in the social care sector
Worksheet 11 – Clients who use the day centre

Bob, care assistant at a day centre   CASE STUDY

My day starts at 8:30am. When I arrive I start to set the room out so that people can sit in groups with others they know. At 9:00am we have a staff briefing. At this meeting the manager talks to us about which clients to expect for the day and also about any special conditions or needs they may have. Our supervisor also talks to us about the programme for the day and makes sure that we know who is responsible for which activities.

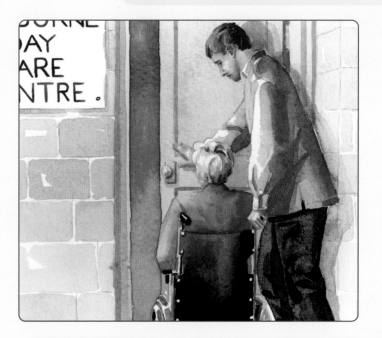

A care assistant needs practical skills to help him in his job

At 10:00am the first people start arriving in the social service buses. I go out and help to wheel in some of the clients who are in wheelchairs. I help them off with their coats and make sure they are sitting comfortably with their friends and get them a cup of coffee or tea. By 11:00am all the groups have arrived and they are busily chatting to one another.

I join each group and read out the lunch menu to them. I ask each of them what they would like but I make sure they know what choices they have first. When all the lunch orders have been taken one of the care assistants starts a quiz for the whole group. We take turns to do this.

At lunchtime I help the clients to the table and make sure they all have the meals they ordered. One lady needs feeding. I ask her what she would like to eat first and tell her what I have on the spoon. The feeding takes some time as she cannot swallow very quickly. I try to make sure I do not spill food down her chin or on her clothes. This helps maintain her dignity.

When clients ask, I take them to the toilet. I make sure that the door is not left wide open. I stand where I can hear them calling but give them enough space to maintain their dignity. When the clients are settled in the community room again after lunch, a game of bingo is organised for those that want to join in. I sit with some, and help them to find the numbers as they are called.

After the bingo I help the group of people that I am responsible for. Someone wants me to help them write a letter. One lady likes knitting, but she is always dropping stitches and cannot pick them up, so I help with this. Another person wants to talk to me about a problem that is worrying him. The afternoon seems to go fairly quickly.

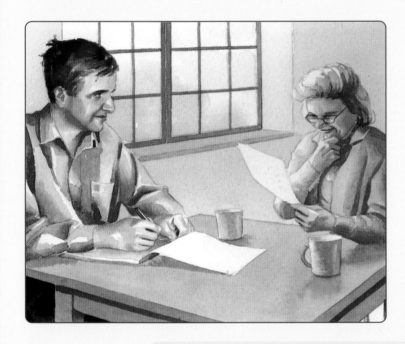

Helping the clients to make the most of their visit

We have tea at 2:45pm and then there is community singing. The clients like to sing some of the 'old' songs. At 3:30pm the transport comes to take them home. I then have to do my record keeping.

I already have an NVQ at level 2 but I am now taking my NVQ in Care at Level 3, while I am working. I go to college one day each week.

35 What skills and qualities is Bob using to meet the needs of the people attending the day centre?

36 How would Bob's work be different if he worked in a residential home?

Jobs in early years settings

> **Word check**
>
> **life experience** – knowing about the wider world after being in school or college.

There is a wide range of jobs that involve looking after children. In many of these jobs, however, a person over the age of 18 is preferred, someone who has some **life experience**.

This is because caring for children can be very demanding and also carries a great deal of responsibility.

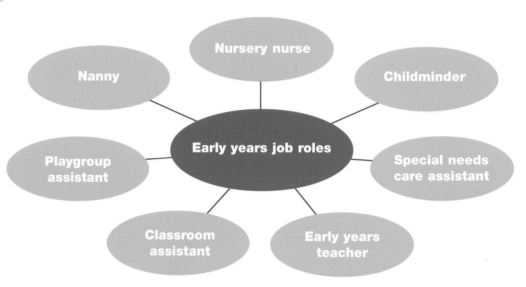

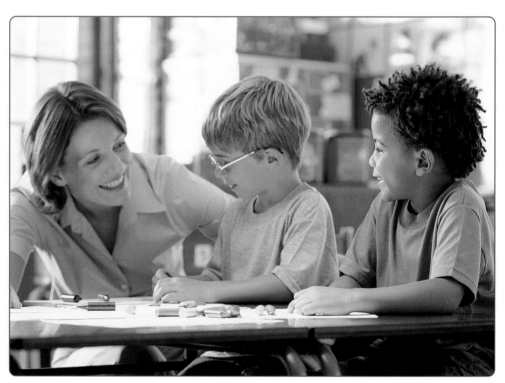

Helping children to develop can be a very rewarding job

Early years training

Training for jobs in early years is varied. One of the most common **routes** for training is to study an NVQ in Child Care or Early Years which often means attending one or two days a week at a local college while the rest of the time is spent getting actual on-the-job experience in looking after children.

Another route is to follow a one or two year college course in order to widen knowledge, skills and understanding of the subject of child development. Courses such as OCR National and Firsts or BTEC National and Firsts aim to equip a person to work in child care environments.

A large number of people who want to work with children follow a course leading to a CACHE Diploma or a Diploma in Nursery Nursing. Nursery nurses are employed, for example, in a hospital, a school or a day nursery. There is no **minimum** age to be a nursery nurse. Having a qualification and some experience of working with children, such as regular babysitting, is most useful. Having a knowledge of First Aid is also helpful.

Anyone under 17 years age, who is working with children, must be supervised at all times by a registered person. To work in a supervisory role, the registered person must have a Level 3 qualification, such as a CACHE Diploma, OCR National in Early Years, BTEC National in Early Years or Level 3 NVQ in Early Years Care and Education.

Word check	✓

route – way of getting somewhere, for example, to a job; a pathway.

Word check	✓

minimum – least or lowest.

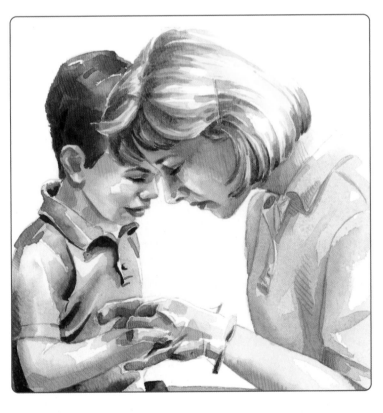

A nursery nurse needs skills in First Aid

Early years settings have a different set of principles and values than those used in health and social care settings. These values can be found in Appendix 9, on page 272.

Appendix 9, see page 272

(T) Worksheet 8 – Finding out about jobs in early years
Worksheet 20 – The values of care in early years settings

Anita, nursery nurse

CASE STUDY

My main job role is to take responsibility for children at the nursery. We take children from three to five years of age. We supervise their play and make sure they are safe. At lunchtime we help them to eat the food that they have brought with them. We have story time and a singalong, as well as lots of creative activities for the children to do at the nursery.

I am working towards an NVQ in Child Care at Level 3 to add to the Nursery Nurse Diploma I got at the local college.

I arrive at work around 8:00am and work through until 4:00pm. Most of the children stay with us for the whole day, but some leave at lunchtime. Most of the children's parents are at work and we look after the children while they are away. We have to be quite sure that we know what each individual child is allowed to do and to eat. We also have to be sure that we have a contact number for the parents in case of an emergency. The children's names and family records are kept on computer, but only two of us can access the information.

There is a short staff meeting to sort out who will supervise the various activities during the day. After the meeting we get out all the equipment and activities ready for when the children arrive. The last children usually arrive around 9:00am.

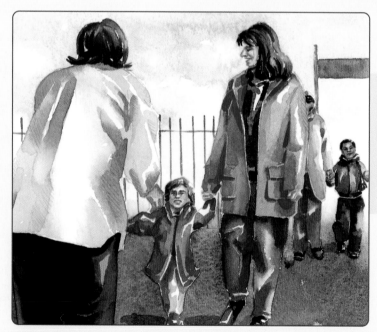

We greet each child in our group individually and make sure we have asked the parent about any special things that have happened or they want us to do. As the children arrive a register is kept so that we know exactly which children are in the building. The parents know that they must actually hand the child to a member of staff and not just leave them to play.

Each child and parent is greeted on arrival

At 9:30am we all get together and greet one another. We have to make sure that the cultural needs of each child are observed. We have different poems and short sayings read out each day during the greeting. This session usually lasts for ten minutes.

Activity time is next. Some children like to paint, some stick and glue, some will colour. Each helper or nursery nurse supervises an activity. We make sure there are lots of different materials from a range of cultures, for the children to use.

At 11:00am there is a drinks break. The children sit in a circle and have a drink and a piece of fruit.

At 11:15am we have story time or singing. This is led by one of the staff, while the children join in and take part in the actions or mime.

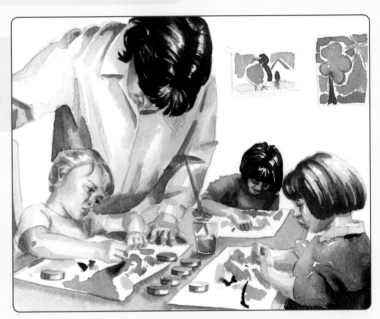

Children love the feel of paint

Before lunch we have 'large' equipment or 'outdoor activities', which means the slide and trampoline are brought out and all the big tractors and cars. The children can go outside if they wish. Sometimes we organise a walk to the park to find things for the 'interest table'.

Quiet music is played after lunch to help the children relax. Each day a tune from a different culture is played.

The children can choose which activity table they sit at during the afternoon. Some activities are different from those provided in the morning. Sometimes we have some finger painting, cooking, or papier-mâché work for the older ones.

Around 3:30pm we have a singalong for five minutes before the free play at the end of the day. Staff try to talk to the parent of each child in their group as they arrive to tell them how they got on.

I enjoy working with the children. It is very satisfying to watch them develop and become more independent and confident.

37 What skills and qualities is Anita using?

Job roles of other care workers in early years settings

We shall now look at the day-to-day tasks of other care workers in early years settings.

Childminder

A childminder should be registered with the local authority social services department. The local authority checks that the childminder's own home has suitable facilities for the children. A childminder must be at least 21 years of age before they can register with the local authority.

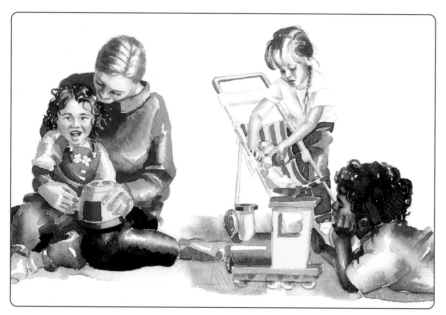

A childminder looks after a small number of children, usually while the parents are working, or if the parent wants to spend some **quality time** with another of their children. The parent may have regular appointments because of a health problem and is unable to take the children, so arranges for a childminder to care for them.

The childminder provides a range of toys for the children to play with and will probably play with the children some of the time. She may take them for a walk or visit a public park or play area.

The childminder is caring for children in her own home

38 How does being a childminder differ from working with children in a day nursery?

Claire, playgroup assistant　　　CASE STUDY

I work in a playgroup and help to supervise the children. I would like to be a playgroup leader when I have more experience and I have agreed to go on some courses with the PLA (or PSLA, Pre-school Learning Alliance) to help prepare me for this. I am taking an NVQ in Child Care but I didn't need a qualification to do this job.

I was invited to take the job after completing work experience. I helped at the playgroup one day a week for 12 weeks. I really enjoyed the work and got on well with the staff. At the playgroup I talk to the children while they are playing or making things. They have very good imaginations and often make up stories about what they are doing.

39 How can a person become a playgroup assistant?

Bret, early years teacher

I studied for three years to get a degree and then trained for a further year to get a teaching certificate (PGCE). I teach the reception class at the local village school. Children learn through play so quite a lot of the teaching I do is by using play activities. The day is structured though and the children have to learn to fit into the pattern of a normal school day.

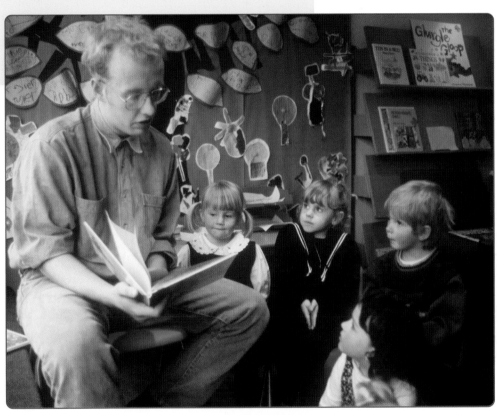

Keeping the attention of young children can be hard

Job roles

Have you read about any jobs that you would like to do? In the activities that follow you will look more closely at some jobs.

A1 Read the case study again for Anita, the nursery nurse on pages 68–69.

- Draw up a table showing FIVE main tasks carried out during her day.

- For each task list TWO skills needed.

A2 How is a childminder's role different from that of a nursery nurse?

A3 Find out TWO different ways for a person to become a qualified nursery nurse.

A4 Explain how a teacher can meet the needs of the children in their group. What effect is having their needs met likely to have on the children?

The values of care

Getting started

All services in health, social care and early years aim to help people to develop and maintain their independence. People who organise care services have to keep a balance between being involved in people's lives or not. When professional care workers give their services to people they apply the values that are an essential part of all care practice.

In this section we shall consider:

- how care workers promote anti-discriminatory practice
- how confidentiality of information is maintained by care workers
- how people's rights to dignity, independence and health and safety are promoted when caring for clients
- how to protect clients from abuse
- how to promote effective communication and relationships between care workers and clients
- how to provide individualised care
- the ways in which the values that underpin care are integrated into codes of practice, policies, procedures and employment contracts of care organisations.

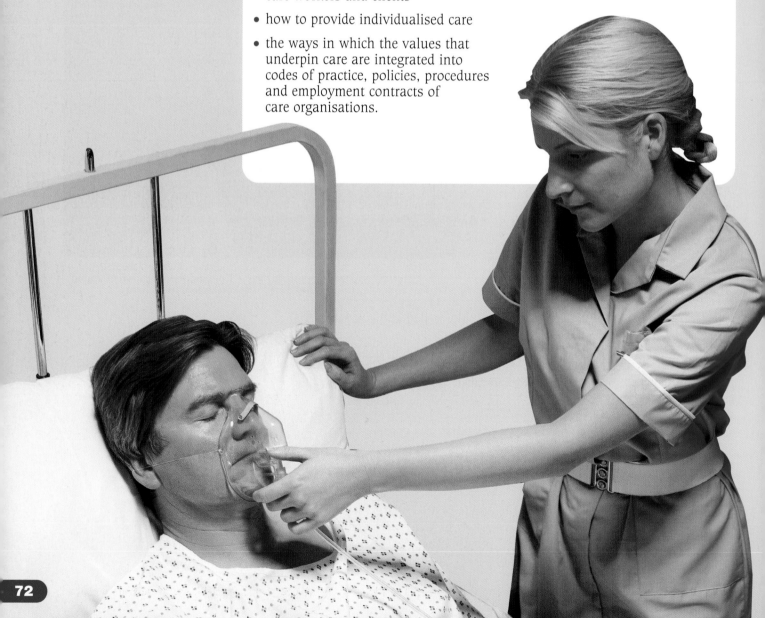

Values that care workers promote through their work

The **values** of care work are centred on ideas about human rights. That is the **rights** to which all individuals are entitled. These rights are given by law through legislation passed in the United Kingdom.

The values of care are way of putting the legislation into practice. It is the way that care workers behave towards individuals when they are caring for them.

> **Word check** ✓
> **rights** – what is due to us.
> **values** – worth or standards.

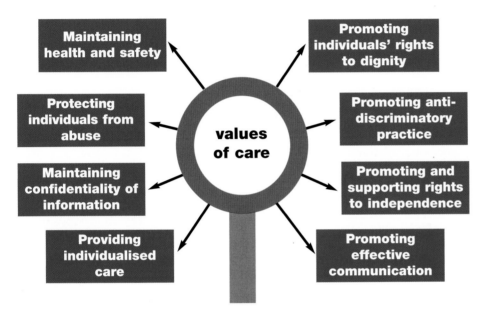

- Maintaining health and safety
- Promoting individuals' rights to dignity
- Protecting individuals from abuse
- Promoting anti-discriminatory practice
- **values of care**
- Promoting and supporting rights to independence
- Maintaining confidentiality of information
- Providing individualised care
- Promoting effective communication

The values that underpin all professional care

If we value a person we want the best for them. We should treat them as we would want to be treated ourselves. A care worker wants to act in 'the best interest of the client' and will, therefore, make sure that in everything they do, they show that they 'value' that person.

40 How could you show a client with Alzheimer's disease that they are valued?

> **Word check** ✓
> **discrimination** – to show bias, or intolerance.
> **gender** – denotes sex, male or female.

Promoting anti-discriminatory practice

Discrimination occurs when a person (or a group of people) is treated unfairly or not given equal treatment. For example, an employer who refuses to give a job of nursery nurse to a male, even though he is the best person for the job, would be discriminating against the person because of his **gender**.

It is important that all care workers take an anti-discriminatory approach in their day-to-day tasks. (In other words they should not discriminate against any person.) In this way, they are applying the values of care.

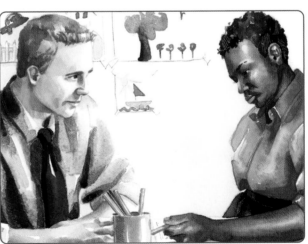

Not all nursery nurses are female

 Worksheet 21 – Values of care in health and social care settings

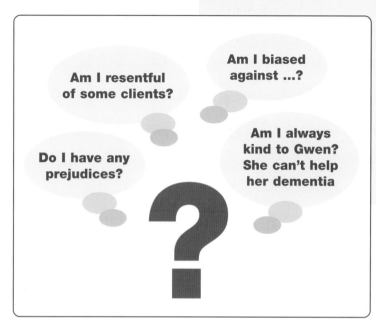

What do I think about …?

Am I resentful of some clients?

Am I biased against …?

Do I have any prejudices?

Am I always kind to Gwen? She can't help her dementia

?

How could care workers prevent discrimination occurring in care settings?

Care workers need to ensure that their own attitudes are non-discriminatory. They need to ask themselves questions to make sure that they are free from prejudices.

They need to ask themselves if they have any hostile feelings or attitudes towards other people. They have to be careful not to make any unfair **judgements** about the people for whom they are caring. They must not **stereotype** individuals.

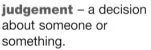

Word check

judgement – a decision about someone or something.

stereotype – to consider all people of a particular group as being the same.

Stereotyping | CASE STUDY

A nurse in the accident and emergency department greets a 20-year-old male who has had a motorcycling accident. The man begins to shout at the nurse and swears. The nurse is forced to call for help because the young man continues to shout and use bad language.

If this man's behaviour leads the nurse to believe that all 20-year-old men who ride motorbikes will act in the same way, she is 'stereotyping' that group of people. Not all 20-year-old motorcyclists would act in this way under the same circumstances.

41 What groups might be stereotyped because of their appearance?

What sort of people are discriminated against?

People who may be treated unfairly or unequally are:

- women
- older people
- people who are physically disabled
- people with learning difficulties
- people who have mental health problems
- people from different cultures or religions, for example, ethnic minorities
- people who have different sexual preferences (lesbian women and gay men).

Discrimination can be in the form of verbal, emotional or physical **abuse**. Emotional abuse is where a person is made to feel that they are not valued. Social abuse, such as not speaking to a person could make them feel **isolated**.

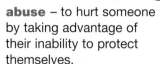

Word check

abuse – to hurt someone by taking advantage of their inability to protect themselves.

isolated – alone; cut off.

Finding out about discrimination ACTIVITY

Have you ever experienced discrimination? If you have you will know how it feels. These activities will help you to understand what discrimination is and how it affects people.

A1 These terms are sometimes used to describe different types of discrimination: *racism, ageism, homophobia* and *disablism*. People may find they are discriminated against because of their *religion* or *health status*.

- Find out what type of discrimination is being shown in each of the words in italics.

A2 Produce a poster that could be used when training care workers to show them how to apply anti-discriminatory practice when caring for clients.

A3 How would you challenge discriminatory practice if you witnessed it happening?

A4 A person has been discriminated against in a care home because of their colour. How do you think the person would feel?

> **Word check**
>
> **confidentiality** – keeping information to oneself.

Maintaining confidentiality

What is **confidentiality**? It means not telling anyone else what a client has said to a care worker. It also means not showing one person's personal notes or computer records to others. Confidentiality means not giving information to anyone else unless there is a very good reason to do so.

To maintain confidentiality puts the values of care into practice because the care worker is acting in the best interest of the client.

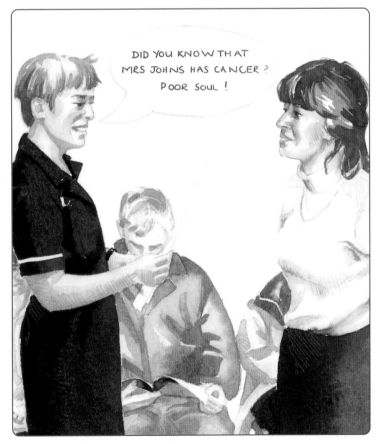

Is this acceptable behaviour?

42 How can a care worker prevent clients from reading other client's notes?

Breaching confidentiality

Are there any occasions when it is right to break confidentially in a care setting? There are only three main reasons for sharing confidential information with another person. These are:

- if someone has said that they are going to harm themselves
- if someone has said they intend to harm another person
- if someone has said they plan to be (or have been) involved in a criminal offence.

If any of these situations arises then the information is only passed to the 'named' or responsible person in the care setting. This person will know how best to deal with the situation and will take the correct action.

It is very easy to break confidentiality when chatting to a friend or **colleague**. Talking about a client to another colleague, by name, loudly enough for people in the waiting room to hear is one example. Another example is going home and saying, "You'll never guess what Tom said today. He ...". The care worker has given the name of the client and broken confidentiality. It is important to refer to individuals in such a way that they cannot be **identified**.

 43 Why is maintaining confidentiality important?

Another way that confidentiality can be broken is by passing information on from one client to another.

> **Word check**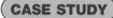
>
> **colleague** – person you work with.
> **identify** – recognise.

Acorns Residential Home ■ CASE STUDY

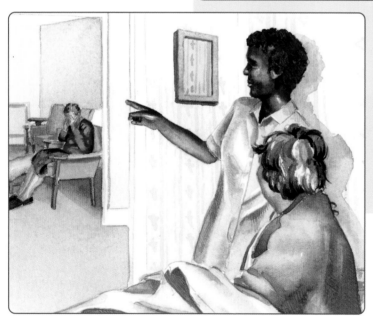

Is nothing private?

Sarah is a care assistant at Acorns Residential Home. She is getting Gwen up in the morning. She tells Gwen, "Come on Gwen, lets get you up. I think you need to go straight to the lounge. Mary is in there looking very down. She's had a phone call from her niece Jackie, and I think she will need someone to talk to."

When Gwen talks to Mary it will be obvious that she knows about the telephone call. Mary will not know how much information Sarah has told Gwen about what was said during the call and may feel that she can no longer **trust** Sarah.

Trust is the basis of any **relationship**, particularly when caring for people. If a client feels that their trust has been broken they will not be so willing to share things in the future.

If a care worker puts confidential information onto the computer it is important that no information is keyed in that breaches the **Data Protection Act**. It is also essential that access to computer records is **restricted** and that only a few named people have the password for the confidential personal and medical records.

44 How does the Data Protection Act protect clients?

Word check

trust – having confidence in a person.

Word check

relationship – two or more people forming a special bond.

Word check

Data Protection Act – law that is to do with informaton that is kept about clients.

restricted – only seen by those who have permission, with a limited number of people having access.

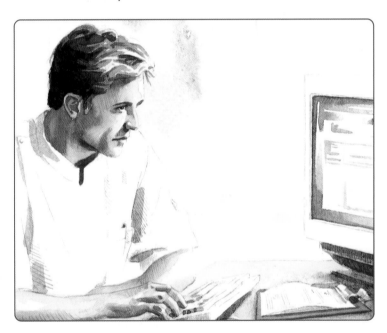

Will this information be kept confidential?

Promoting and supporting the rights of individuals

What are people's rights? People have the right to:

- be different
- have freedom from discrimination
- confidentiality
- choice
- dignity
- effective communication
- safety and security.

Word check ✓

decision – a resolution,
an outcome.
informed – having
knowledge.

Making choices

Applying the values of care and promoting client rights means that the care worker makes sure that the client is given the opportunity to make choices. Choices can vary from major **decisions** about the treatment they wish to have, to smaller decisions about choosing the clothes they wear and the food they eat. In order to make choices the client needs to be given information so that they can make **informed** decisions.

For example, the consultant at the hospital, tells Ahmed that he has cancer of the bowel and that he should have an operation. Ahmed needs to know how long the operation will take; what are his chances of recovery; what are the likely after-effects; and whether there are any alternatives to surgery, such as chemotherapy. Ahmed cannot make any decisions or choices until he has all the information.

Word check ✓

independent – able to do
things without help.

Imagine you are a care assistant in a client's home. You are helping to get the client dressed and give them breakfast. To apply the values of care the client should be allowed to choose what to wear and what to eat. Before they can choose they must know what there is to choose from. This may take a little more time, but by taking this approach the client will feel empowered and more **independent**. The care worker would then be applying the values of care as they are acting in the best interest of the client.

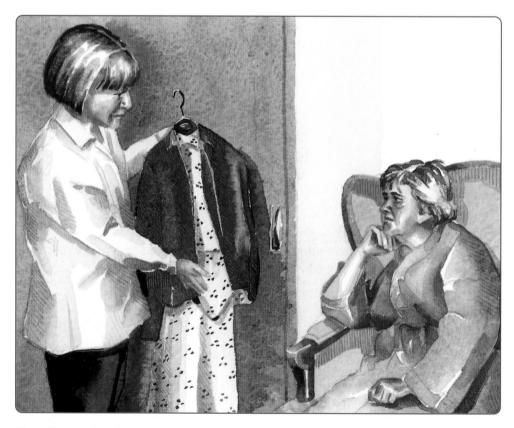

You will wear these!

Maintaining dignity

Imagine Ahmed has had an operation to remove part of his bowel. The nurse wants to check the wound and put on a clean dressing. How can this be done and maintain Ahmed's **dignity**? To allow Ahmed to keep his dignity, the nurse has to apply the values of care by:

- drawing the curtains around Ahmed's bed

- explaining to Ahmed what he is going to do

- asking Ahmed if he wants to ask about any part of the procedure

- uncovering only the area that needs attention and making sure other private areas are not exposed

- talking in a low voice so that others in the ward will not overhear

- making sure Ahmed is dressed and comfortable before pulling back the curtains.

By applying the values of care in this way the nurse has maintained Ahmed's dignity and **privacy**.

Let us think about a care assistant feeding a client who is unable to feed herself. How will the values of care be applied in this situation?

The care assistant should:

- prepare the client by sitting her in a comfortable position

- explain the actions he is going to take

- ask the person what she would like to eat first

- explain how he is going to do the feeding

- put very small amounts of food on the spoon and place it carefully in the client's mouth

- allow the client enough time to chew the food before putting in the next portion

- clear up any spillages using a serviette or cloth, making sure that he explains what he is doing.

The client's dignity is maintained as the care assistant shows respect and consults the client during each step in the process. The care worker applies the values of care because his actions show that he is acting in the client's best interest.

Word check
dignity – self-respect.

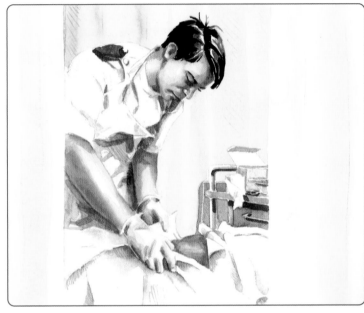

Maintaining the patient's dignity is important

Word check ✓
privacy – being private.

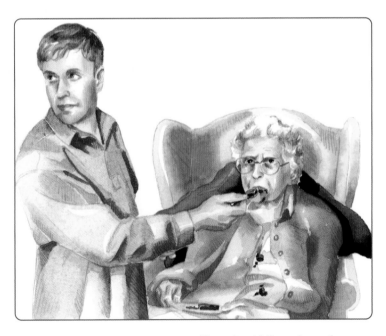

How should the values of care be applied in this situation?

Acknowledging personal beliefs and identity

Care workers need to be aware that a person from another culture, or who has different religious beliefs, may need to have special arrangements made. This could be to enable them to pray at a time that their religion requires. The person may not want to eat the usual food that is provided at meal times and therefore, a choice of food, that they are able to eat, should be available.

Some cultural customs have rules about the relationship between men and women, and about what the members of each sex can and cannot do. For example, female clients may have to be treated by a female doctor or consultant. A female client may need to have an older relative with them when they are having a consultation, as this may be part of their tradition. In some cultures, major decisions are taken only by the male head of the family. So if, for example, a woman needs an operation, her husband or father would have to give permission. Care workers must be sensitive to these issues and need to find out about a client's beliefs. They should be prepared to offer suitable choices and care routines.

Anti-discriminatory care practice means making sure that people have the same chances or opportunities in care. For example, a person over 75 should not be thought of as being less important, because of their age, when considering their treatment and care. They should be given the same opportunities for treatment and care as a younger person with a similar condition or illness.

In early years services, such as day nurseries, children should have toys that reflect a range of cultures. Stories that are read to children should not be drawn just from one country but from a variety of sources.

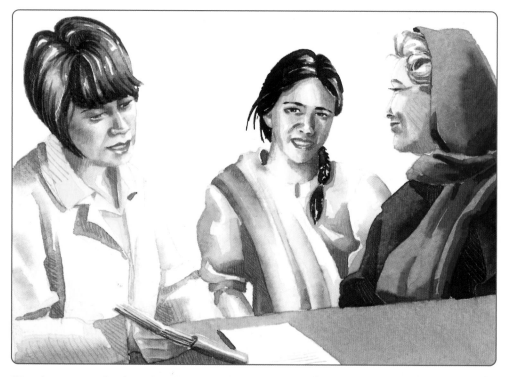

Showing respect for the cultural wishes of the client

What happens in care settings?

Employers in care settings try to ensure that discrimination and prejudice do not occur. Often, policies are in place to help protect the people who use the settings. Everything is done to promote the values that underpin care. Try to investigate for yourselves how this is done.

A1 Make arrangements to visit a care setting (you must get your teacher's permission first).

A2 Produce a list of questions to ask during the visit about:

- how confidentiality is maintained in the care setting
- how people's rights are promoted
- how clients' dignity is maintained
- how clients are encouraged to make choices
- how the care workers help clients maintain their independence.

A3 Trial your questionnaire to make sure it will give you the answers you need.

A4 Visit the care setting to gather the information. If you are unable to visit you may be able to invite a care worker to your school.

A5 Collate the information you have collected.

A6 Present the information using some of the following methods: pie charts, graphs, line diagrams, bar charts, written information.

Word check

vulnerable – at risk of harm.

Word check

power – having control, or a hold over someone.

Protecting individuals from abuse

Abuse can take many forms and can be used against any service user who is unable to protect themselves. Abuse can be physical, emotional or social. Those who are most **vulnerable** are older people, children and people who have a disability including both physical disabilities and learning difficulties.

Preventing abuse

Working as a team in a care setting can help to prevent abuse. A team shares and talks about the things that happen and so abuse is less likely to arise.

Abuse is likely to happen when people are overworked, or do not have enough time to do their job properly. Or it could happen if a person has their own prejudices about certain people or things. Anxiety and worry can also contribute to people being abused. Sometimes a care worker abuses a client because they feel it gives them **power** over the person.

In a care situation abuse, if spotted, should be reported straight away to a supervisor or manager so that action can be taken immediately.

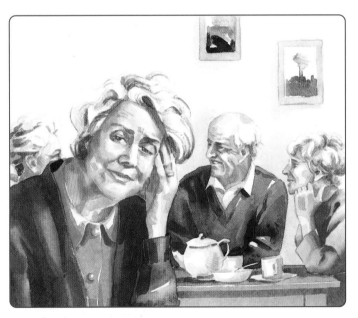

Ida has been isolated. This is a form of abuse.

David
CASE STUDY

David is 80. He cannot look after himself properly. His son shouts and waves his fists at David because he is angry. The house is messed up again. He only tidied it up two days before. He tells David he 'should be locked away in a home'.

45 How do you think David feels?

Judith
CASE STUDY

Judith is seven. She has been locked in her room by her stepmum. She would like to play with the other children but her stepmum has told her that no one would want to play with her as she is too stupid and ugly.

46 What effect is this treatment likely to have on Judith?

Steve
CASE STUDY

Steve lives in a residential home. His room is on the second floor. The lift has broken down and he cannot get down to the lounge for the concert. The staff tell him he will have to stay in his room as no one has time to carry him downstairs. Steve feels left out.

47 What type of abuse is being shown to Steve?

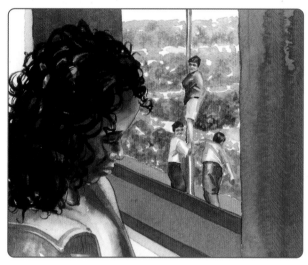

Judith is not allowed out

Ling
CASE STUDY

Ling is 68 years of age but she has learning difficulties. She lives in a residential home with other adults, some of whom have learning difficulties. Ling cannot get to and from the toilet without help. She has been waiting for over half an hour for someone to help her back to the lounge.

Dealing with abuse
ACTIVITY

How do you think you would feel if you found yourself in any of the case studies given above? Let us think about each situation more closely.

A1 In each case a person is being abused. For each situation:

- state the type of abuse that is happening
- explain how the abuse could be prevented
- explain the effect of the abuse on the person.

A2 Describe the action that should be taken by care workers if they see clients being abused.

A3 How could abuse be prevented in a care setting? How would the methods you suggest empower the clients?

Promoting effective communication and relationships

There are many different types of relationship. From a very early age until the time we die, the main feature of a successful relationship is sharing and being able to support one another. This is particularly important when working in care settings. Everyone is more effective when they share workloads, information and ideas. Clients, too, want to share their problems and their feelings in a successful relationship.

A client may be **dependent** on care workers. They rely on the care worker to treat them as a valued person. They trust the care worker not to do anything that will harm them. This may give the care worker a feeling of power because they know that the person has to rely on them. In an ideal client-carer relationship there is a **balance** of power, with the care worker respecting the rights of the client and applying the values of care.

Word check

dependent – needing help from others, not being able to do things for oneself.

Word check

balance – in the correct proportions.

Verbal skills

Effective communication should be at the heart of any relationship. This means that care workers need to be aware of the skill that they need when communicating orally with clients. What are these skills?

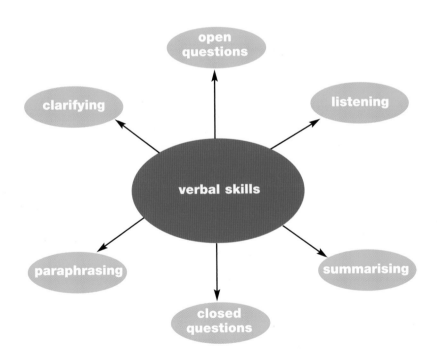

Word check

non-verbal communication – not using speech, but using body language, such as smiling.

Non-verbal skills

Non-verbal communication can also be important when caring for clients. Sometimes this is called 'body language'. We all use body language when we are with other people. This could be in the form of a smile, or hand gestures, or facial expressions, for example.

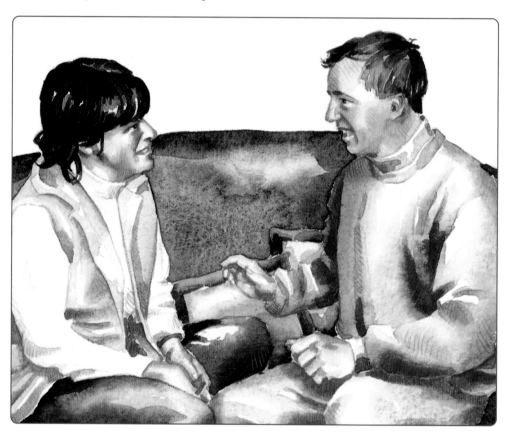

Body language can help conversation

Word check

Makaton – a type of sign language.

Braille – a method of reading by running fingers over raised symbols.

Word check

actively – being involved.

People who are deaf may use sign language to help them communicate with others. People who are deaf and have other severe learning difficulties may use **Makaton**, another kind of signing. Those who are blind may communicate with others by using **Braille**.

When we communicate with others we should also remember that they need to understand what we are saying and we need to understand their responses. We might use the skills shown in the illustration on page 83 to aid understanding.

Listening is a very important part of communicating. We have to train ourselves to listen **actively**, that is, to follow the whole of the conversation with interest. We can confirm that we have understood by clarifying or paraphrasing.

Getting on with people ## ACTIVITY

How well do you get on with people? Can you communicate well with others? If you are going to work in a care setting or if you are an informal carer at any time in your life, it will be important to communicate effectively with your clients.

A1 Use each of the words in the box below in a sentence to show that you understand their meaning:

> **open question**   **paraphrasing**   **closed question**
>
> **summarising**   **reflecting**   **clarifying**   **active listening**

A2 Look at each of the situations shown in the table. Explain how each situation might affect client-carer relationships.

Situation	Effect on client-carer relationships
Interrupting when the client is telling you something	
Criticising the client in public	
Talking publicly about a letter the client has received that has upset them	

A3 Louisa is in her seventies and has arthritis. A care assistant, Annie, visits her each day to help her with the shopping and some housework.

- Complete the table below to give an example of how Annie could use the skills shown when talking to Louisa.

Skill used by Annie	Example of what she might say
An open question	
A closed question	
Summarising	

Providing individualised care

Word check

individualised – designed for one person.

A client's needs are usually assessed by a social worker, an occupational therapist, or by a GP. When the assessment has been completed a care plan will be drawn up with the client. This care plan will be based on the client's own needs and so it will be **individualised**. There may be a large number of patients or several people living in a residential home, but each will have their own care plan to suit their specific needs. In this way the values of care are being applied and the clients' rights are being promoted as they are being treated as individuals not as a group.

Meeting clients' needs   ACTIVITY

Different methods can be used to find out what clients think about how services meet their needs. Firstly, it is important to find out what their needs are. Then we have to find out how those needs can be met by health, social care and early years services.

A1 Arrange to visit a care setting and find out the needs of THREE clients. If this is not possible, maybe three clients could be invited into school.

* Draw up a questionnaire to find out the needs of each client, and how those needs are being met.

A2 Trial the questionnaire before it is used to check that it will provide the information needed. Adjust the questionnaire if necessary.

A3 Visit the care setting to find out about the needs of THREE clients using the questionnaire.

A4 Collate all the information.

A5 Explain how the service meets the needs of each client.

A6 How are the clients affected by having their needs met?

Codes of practice, policies and procedures

How do codes of practice, policies and procedures help to ensure that the values of care are applied?

Codes of practice

Word check

code of practice – a set of guidelines; a framework within which to work.

Professional care workers are trained to apply the values of care in their work. They are also helped in this, because they are expected to follow a **code of practice**.

Part of the Nursing and Midwifery Council's Code of professional conduct is reproduced on the next page. This is issued to all registered nurses, midwives and health visitors. The Council is the regulatory body responsible for the standards of these professions and it requires members of the professions to practise and conduct themselves within the standards and framework provided by the Code.

Code of professional conduct

As a registered nurse, midwife or health visitor, you are personally accountable for your practice. In caring for patients and clients, you must:

- respect the patient or client as an individual
- obtain consent before you give any treatment or care
- protect confidential information
- cooperate with others in the team
- maintain your professional knowledge and competence
- be trustworthy
- act to identify and minimise risk to patients and clients.

These are the shared values of all the United Kingdom health care regulatory bodies.

5 **As a registered nurse, midwife or health visitor, you must protect confidential information.**

5.1 You must treat information about patients and clients as confidential and use it only for the purposes for which it was given. As it is impractical to obtain consent every time you need to share information with others, you should ensure that patients and clients understand that some information may be made available to other members of the team involved in the delivery of care. You must guard against breaches of confidentiality by protecting information from improper disclosure at all times.

5.2 You should seek patients' and clients' wishes regarding the sharing of information with their family and others. When a patient or client is considered incapable of giving permission, you should consult relevant colleagues.

5.3 If you are required to disclose information outside the team that will have personal consequences for patients or clients, you must obtain their consent. If the patient or client withholds consent, or if consent cannot be obtained for whatever reason, disclosures may be made only where:

- they can be justified in the public interest (usually where disclosure is essential to protect the patient or client or someone else from the risk of significant harm)
- they are required by law or by order of a court.

5.4 Where there is an issue of child protection, you must act at all times in accordance with national and local policies.

Extracts from the Nursing and Midwifery Council's code of professional conduct

Word check

framework – structure or boundaries.

A code of practice is a guide for the care worker to how they should act when they are caring for clients. It provides a **framework** within which they work. The values of care and the code of practice work together to protect the client and to promote their interests.

A code of practice informs a care worker how to behave when caring for a client. Nurses, midwives and health visitors follow a code of professional conduct. See the extracts on page 87.

This code of practice very closely matches the values in care as it requires care workers to show respect, maintain dignity and avoid doing anything that will harm the client. Any nurse, midwife or health visitor has to follow this code of practice. It applies right across the United Kingdom, not just to one organisation.

There are other codes of practice that apply across different types of care settings. One is 'Home Life, a code of practice for residential homes'. This of course applies to all residential homes in the United Kingdom. Another code of practice is the SEN (Special Educational Needs) code of practice which is applied across all UK educational establishments, to give guidance on helping children with special needs.

A code of practice is not law. It may be produced as a result of a law. It is a set of **standards** that helps to maintain and support clients and to provide a guide to care workers' responsibilities.

Word check

standards – a level of quality.

Codes of practice are often closely linked to the values of care and include some of the values in the 'good practice' they set out.

The table gives some examples of how this happens.

Code of practice	The values of care
No action is detrimental to the patient	Promote health and safety
Foster the independence of the client and respect their involvement in the planning and delivery of their care	Promote and support individuals' rights to independence and provide individualised care
Act in a manner to promote and safeguard the interest and well-being of patients	Protect the individual from abuse Promote anti-discriminatory practice
Protect all confidential information concerning patients	Maintain confidentiality of information

Codes of practice and the values of care have common aims and complement one another. They work together for the benefit and support of the patient.

Policies

Often when a code of practice has been formed, policies are written. A policy is based on sections or parts of the code of practice. For example, a health and safety policy should identify who is responsible for the safety of the setting and the people in it.

Other policies might include a policy for the employment of care staff or a policy for moving and handling clients.

A policy applies to a particular care setting or a group of care settings. It tells the care workers how to approach specific tasks. It should explain in detail, for example, how to move and handle clients. The policies affect and influence the procedures that are carried out in a care setting. In other words, it demonstrates 'the way things are done'.

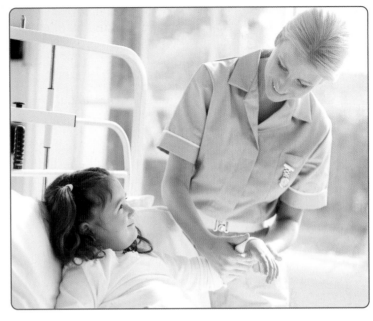

Feeling safe and secure

Procedures

Care settings have **procedures** that must be followed. For example, there is usually a procedure to follow when maintenance staff are seeking access to a nursing or residential home. There is normally a procedure to follow when a person has had an accident, for example, an accident report book may need to be completed.

All policies and procedures aim to look after the best interests of the clients. The staff in a care setting would want to ensure that the values of care are applied in all its activities. Treating the client as an individual who has rights, and wanting to respect their individuality, is important in any care setting.

> **Word check** ✓
>
> **procedure** – course of action that must be followed.

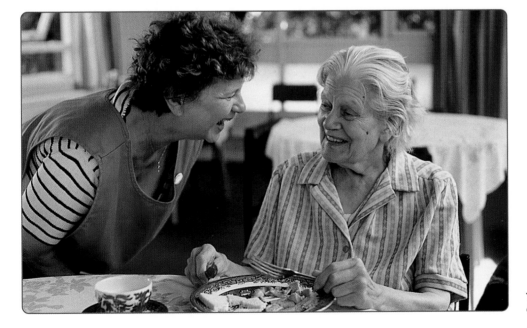

The best interests of the client are being promoted

 Unit 1 assignment

2 Promoting health and well-being

Contents

About this unit

You will learn about:

- definitions of health and well-being
- common factors that affect health and well-being and the different effects they can have on individuals and groups across the lifespan
- methods used to measure an individual's physical health
- ways of promoting and supporting health improvement for an individual or small group.

The knowledge that you will gain from this unit will help you to look after your own health and well-being and understand ways of promoting health and well-being for others.

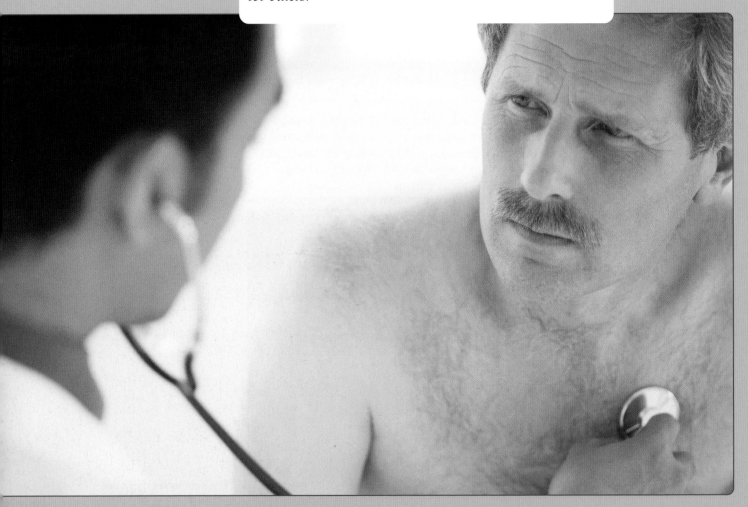

Introducing this unit

How do you know if you are healthy and well? We all want to be healthy but do we know when we are? Personal health is a subject that is of interest to many people. We can describe being healthy as being free from physical illnesses and disease and avoiding stress. Keeping physically fit and mentally alert is also part of being healthy. We will learn that well-being is how people feel about themselves. Feeling good about yourself is an important part of keeping healthy.

In this unit we will be looking at the factors that help us to stay healthy. These include, for example, diet, exercise and lifestyle. We shall also find out about the different risks that can affect our health. Activities like smoking, drinking and unprotected sex can give us a higher risk of illness and disease. Understanding these risks is an important part of this unit.

We will learn how we can measure health, by looking at the links between weight, height and blood pressure. These links will help us see how monitoring can lead to improvements in individual health.

We will also examine ways to improve our health and how we feel. To do this we will look at health promotion information produced by various health organisations. This will allow us to plan improvements to our own and other people's health.

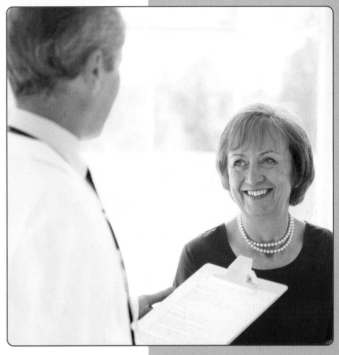

Looking and feeling good

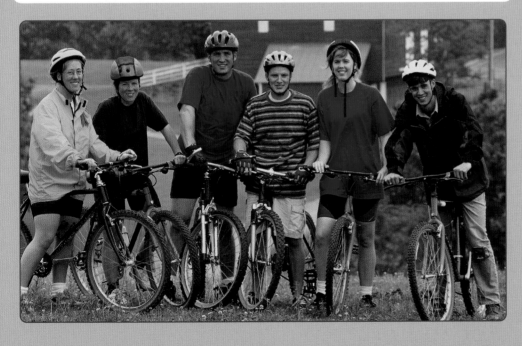

Exercise helps to keep us healthy and happy

Understanding health and well-being

Getting started

What is health and well-being?

Health and well-being can mean different things for different people. This is because different factors affect our health and well-being.

In this section you will:

- look at what people consider to be good health
- understand how well-being is affected
- understand the difference between disease and illness
- look at how our changing needs affect our health and well-being
- look at how ideas about health and well-being have changed over the years.

Planning to help us stay healthy

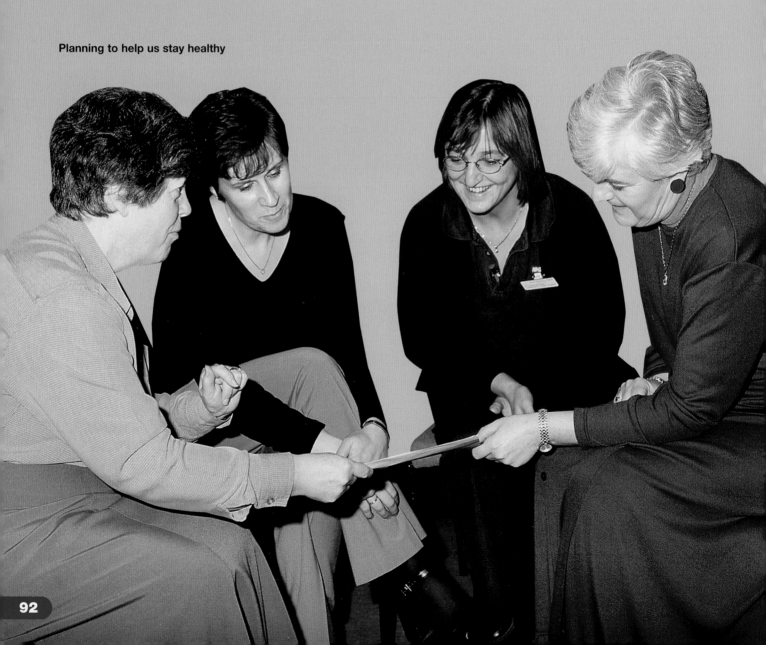

Good health

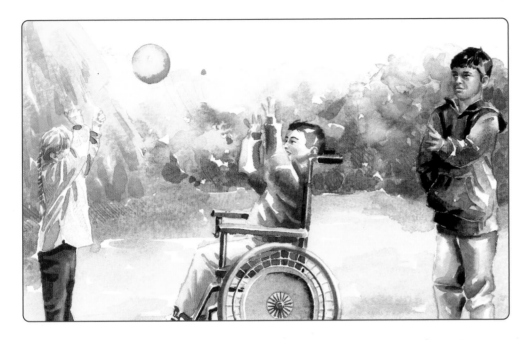

Being physically impaired does not mean that you are unhealthy

Good health means different things to different people. This is because there are different ways of looking at health. Some people think of themselves as healthy if they have no illness or disease.

If you have a **positive** view of health you see things in a different light. You look at everything that you can do well, for example, being able to walk and run, having a full and active life, being fit and feeling well.

Whatever approach we take, being healthy is different for each person. People can have various physical conditions that could be considered as poor health. It is still possible to be healthy if you are confined to a wheelchair. Not being able to walk does not make you unhealthy.

Today we like to take an **holistic** view of health and well-being. This means that we look at every part of a person's life. It allows us to look at the bigger picture of all of the events that affect us.

The World Health Organisation gives us a very positive and holistic description of health. Their definition is:

'a state of complete physical, mental and social well-being, not merely the absence of disease and infirmity.'

We can see that this definition involves a broad view of health. It includes physical, mental and social well-being.

1 What is the meaning of the word holistic?

Word check

positive – concentrating on what is good.

Word check

holistic – to look at the whole; to consider the whole person.

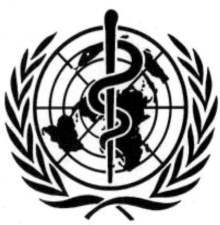

Logo of the World Health Organisation (WHO)

Understanding well-being

If you say to your teacher, 'How are you today?', the chances are that the reply will be, 'Very well, thank you'. This means that they are feeling well in themselves. Well-being is how people feel about themselves. The sense of well-being that a person has is affected by different influences.

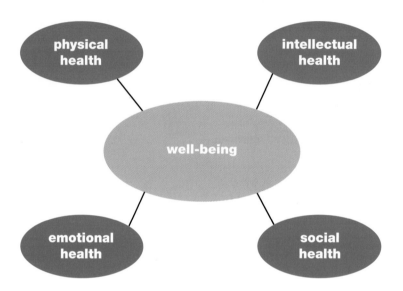

Each area of our lives is affected if we have poor health

The list shows us what can affect our well-being:

* physical health
* intellectual health
* emotional health
* social health.

These are known as **aspects** of health.

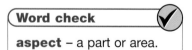
PIES, see page 9

Physical health

Physical health is how our body is **functioning**. If we are fit and healthy we can be said to be in good physical health.

Intellectual health

Intellectual health is our ability to think, learn and make decisions and judgements. Our intellectual health is maintained by everyday activities. We are always learning from changes that happen around us and decisions that we make. Everything that we read, watch and listen to has an effect on our intellectual health.

Word check ✓

aspect – a part or area.

Word check ✓

function – work.

Emotional health

Emotional health involves our ability to understand and recognise our personal feelings. These include happiness, anger and fear, and we show these in different ways. How we feel depends on what is happening around us.

Social health

We are all involved in relationships with other people. Our friends and family often influence the way that we think and feel. We are affected by where we live, our education, our job and how much money we have. All of these can have greater or lesser effects on our well-being.

Mental health

Alongside our physical, intellectual, emotional and social health and well-being we also need to think about our state of mental health.

Mental health is a difficult concept to understand. We can consider it as the ability to cope with our everyday lives. If we can cope with the stress and worries of everyday life without breaking down, we can maintain good mental health. Good mental health allows us to think clearly and make correct decisions.

2 What is your definition of health and well-being?

We can now see that well-being can be a **complex** subject. All of its **components** are events that we experience, often on a daily basis.

> **Word check**
>
> **complex** – difficult, or having many functions.

> **Word check**
>
> **component** – a part of.

What is health? (**ACTIVITY**)

A1 Write your own definition about what is meant by 'good health'.

A2 Make a leaflet to explain to people what 'ill-health' is.

A3 You want to find out about a person's health status.

Write EIGHT questions, TWO for each of the following aspects of their health:

- physical

- intellectual

- emotional

- social.

A4 Working in small groups, discuss the questions that you have written. Rewrite any questions that you now feel need changing.

A5 Try out your questions on a member of one of the other groups.

A6 Use the answers that you have been given to show the health status of the person who answered the questions.

A7 What else would you need to ask to get a full health profile for that person? You will need to find out about factors that have had a positive (good) effect on the person, for example, family or education, and factors that have had a bad effect on their health, for example, bullying or lack of money.

Personal health needs

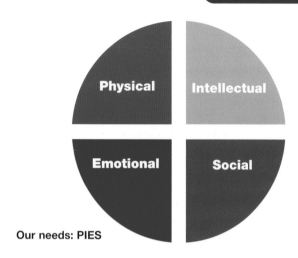

Our needs: PIES

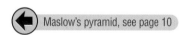
Maslow's pyramid, see page 10

Maslow's pyramid, see page 10

If well-being is how people feel about themselves, who is the best person to judge well-being? The answer is the person themselves. Well-being is underpinned by a collection of personal health needs. Good supportive relationships, food, shelter, warmth and money are just some of things that maintain well-being.

Our needs include **P**hysical, **I**ntellectual, **E**motional and **S**ocial needs.

Turn back to Maslow's pyramid in Unit 1 (see page 10) to remind yourself about our basic needs. Look again at Maslow's way of arranging these needs.

3 What are our basic needs?

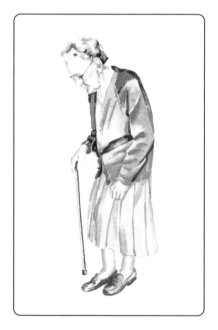

Older people can lose up to seven centimetres in height

The effect of age

Age affects our basic needs. In our early life stages we are very dependent on others. Our dependency on others reduces as we mature. Our health is influenced by various factors. As we get older, our body systems can become weaker and we become more **prone** to disease and illness. Therefore, as we age we change.

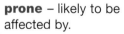

Word check

prone – likely to be affected by.

Disease and illness

Disease and illness show themselves in many forms and it is important to know the difference between the two. Doctors and health care professionals use the words disease and illness in a set way.

Disease

Disease has been described as 'an **observable** physical change in the body's structure'. Or, something that causes a change in the way the body functions.

This means that you can often see the effects and symptoms of a disease. If someone has **chicken pox** you can see the spots. If they have a head cold then you will hear them sneeze and see that they have a red nose. These are known as symptoms and draw your attention to the disease.

4 How many different diseases can you think of in one minute?

Illness

Illness is the term given to the effects that a person feels when they have a disease. This means that the person may complain of feeling unwell. The person who has chicken pox will want to scratch because the spots itch. The person with the head cold will feel unwell and they may have aches and pains. These symptoms cannot always be seen by others, but can be described by the person suffering.

5 What is the difference between illness and disease?

Word check	

observable – something that you can see.

Word check	

chicken pox – a disease that affects mostly children, giving them spots and a fever.

Attitudes to health and well-being

You have probably noticed that **attitudes** to health vary. If we look back in history we can see that people's views of health and well-being have changed over time. While we are fit and well we tend not to worry too much about our health. When something happens to us to make us feel unwell then we begin to think about our condition and to consider just how healthy we really are. At this point sometimes the damage is already done.

Now, various agencies, like the British Heart Foundation, try to raise our awareness of particular health issues. Their aim is to help people focus more on their own health. The idea is to help stop people getting ill by giving advice. If people follow their advice it helps reduce heart disease.

Word check	

attitude – thoughts, views and behaviour.

How can our health be affected? | ACTIVITY

A1 Arrange to talk to a parent about any illnesses that their child has had. Find out how the child's health was affected.

A2 Interview an older person to find out how they see their health status. What are the main factors that have influenced their health status?

A3 Compare the different views you obtained.

A4 Draw conclusions about each person's health status.

Health targets

Health information that care workers provide is often linked to government plans. These plans are intended to help improve the whole nation's health. The idea behind the plans is to persuade people to live a healthier lifestyle. A better diet, more exercise, and drinking and smoking less can make people healthier.

One of the key **objectives** of a government is to set targets. In 1992 a number of national health targets were identified for England. These were published in a government document called The Health of the Nation. The idea was to improve the health of the whole population by the year 2010. After much **research** the government felt that there were health areas where they could make big improvements. Their targeted areas would be:

- coronary heart disease
- **stroke**
- cancers
- HIV and AIDS
- accidents
- mental illness.

Coronary heart disease and stroke

The government had good reasons for selecting these areas. Coronary heart disease and stroke were selected because they are **preventable**. Diet, fitness and lifestyle have a big **influence** on these.

Cancers

Cancers were identified as an increasing danger. They were targeted because many can be:

- prevented
- cured
- controlled.

The aim is to check people who appear to be healthy on a regular basis for early signs of disease. This is known as screening. If a cancer is found they can be given treatment quickly.

Word check

objective – something you set out to do.
research – obtain information.

Word check

stroke – common name for the effects of a broken blood vessel in the brain.

Word check

preventable – stoppable.
influence – an effect on a person.

Screening, see page 121

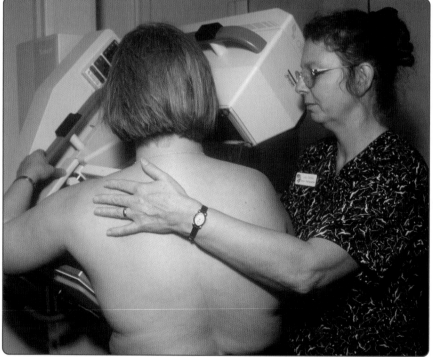

Early detection of any form of cancer can save lives

HIV and AIDS

HIV causing AIDS is proving to be the greatest new threat to the health of the public. There has been a serious spread of this disease in continents such as Africa and the number of cases in the United Kingdom is continuing to rise. The government therefore saw it as a threat that had to be challenged. For more facts about HIV and AIDS, see the data on page 142.

HIV/AIDS data, see page 142

Accidents

We know that accidents are preventable. By making everyone more aware of risks the government could reduce the number of accidents each year. This could lead to huge savings in the health **budget** that could be used to help the health service elsewhere.

Mental illness

Mental illness was targeted because it can affect everyone. By improving services it was felt that the nation's mental health could be improved.

Word check

budget – an amount of money put aside for a certain purpose.

6 Why do you think these targets have been set by the government?

The Health of the Nation plan

These are some of the targets that the government set.

By the year 2000

Health problem	Target
Heart disease and stroke in people under 65	reduced by 40%
Breast cancer deaths in women between the ages of 50 and 64	reduced by 25%

By the year 2005

Health problem	Target
Fatal accidents in children under the age of 15	reduced by 33%
Fatal accidents in young adults	reduced by 25%

By the year 2010

Health problem	Target
Lung cancer deaths in men under the age of 75	reduced by 30%
Lung cancer deaths in women under the age of 75	reduced by 15%

The remaining targets were to cut:

Health problem	Target
Suicide rates	reduced by 15%
Suicide rates in the mentally ill	reduced by 33%
HIV and sexually transmitted disease rates	reduced

Our Healthier Nation

Some improvements were achieved in the 1990s but the government has not given up. The plan has continued and been revised. In 1998 a new plan was introduced called Our Healthier Nation.

The new plan aims to help improve the health and well-being of the most **disadvantaged** and least healthy. It is attempting to improve the areas in which they live.

The new plan tries to address some of the problems that are beyond the control of the general public:

- housing
- the environment
- pollution
- poverty
- crime.

All these factors have an effect on our health and well-being and the government wants to see them given more attention.

7 Who, in the UK, is classed as disadvantaged?

Priority areas

The government wants to help society to tackle these problems. Families, **communities** and local agencies will be the front line in tackling the problems. The government hopes that by providing help the needs of the people can be met.

The problems highlighted in The Health of the Nation have not changed. But there are now four priority areas, with similar aims:

- heart disease and stroke reduced by 33%
- cancer reduced by 20%
- mental illness reduced by 17%
- accidents reduced by 20%.

The government believes that it can make the greatest difference in these areas.

People who have social problems and live in poor **neighbourhoods** are often more at risk from the targeted problems.

8 What are the main problems that are beyond the control of the general public?

Word check

disadvantaged – unable to fulfill basic needs.

Word check

community – group of people living in the same area, or having something in common.

Word check

neighbourhood – area where a group of people live.

Meeting the targets

There is much to be done if these targets are to be met. Health education will focus on three areas:

- schools

- workplaces

- neighbourhoods.

The proposed action should result in children, adults, older people and in fact the whole community, being healthier. The target date is still 2010. As each year passes the state of all our health and well-being should improve!

9 What target would you set if you were developing a health plan for your school or college?

Promoting good health   ACTIVITY

A1 As a group discuss: 'Why is it important for the nation that a government promotes good health for everyone?'

- After the discussion write down your own opinion.

A2 Why do you think health education is an important feature in helping to meet the targets?

A3 One of the government targets is to reduce heart disease and strokes. What additional health and social care services might be needed to help achieve this?

Factors and risks affecting health and well-being

Getting started

Throughout life, a person's health and well-being are affected by a number of different factors, both positive and negative.

In this section we will look at both the positive influences and the risks to health and well-being. For example, we shall think about how to provide a balanced diet and look at the risks we run through poor nutrition.

This section will therefore help you to:

- understand what makes up a balanced diet and the risks associated with a poor diet
- understand the benefits of regular exercise and the health risks of lack of exercise
- look at the value of supportive relationships and the effects of social isolation
- understand why adequate housing and financial resources are important to health and well-being
- understand the need for stimulating work, education and leisure activities, and the negative effects of unemployment
- look at the value of health monitoring and methods of preventing ill-health
- understand the need for risk management and personal safety.

Other risks we shall consider will be those associated with:

- lack of personal hygiene
- having unprotected sex
- environmental pollution.

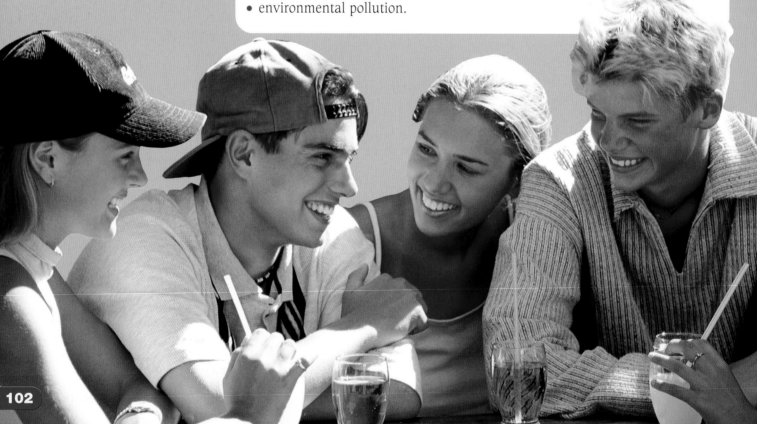

A balanced diet

The food that we eat plays an important role in maintaining our health. An essential part of healthy eating is to balance our diet. By doing this we provide our body with everything that it needs to grow and function. If we have a balanced diet we avoid building up too much stored fat. It also stops our body developing any **deficiencies** from missing essential vitamins and minerals.

So what is a balanced diet? A balanced diet is made up of the following seven essential components:

- protein
- fat
- carbohydrate
- vitamins
- minerals
- water
- fibre.

In a balanced diet, we have these components in the correct amounts or proportions to meet our individual needs.

All of the above contribute to at least one of these functions:

- building, repairing and maintaining the body
- **regulating** body processes and functions
- providing energy.

10 What are the seven essential components in our diet?

> **Word check**
>
> **deficiency** – to have less than is needed.

> **Word check**
>
> **regulate** – control.

> **Word check**
>
> **amino acids** – chemicals that are the building blocks of protein.

Protein

Proteins are used to build our body. When we are children they are very important for building the brain, muscle, skin, blood and other tissues. Proteins also provide the materials needed to repair the cells in our body.

Proteins are made up of chemicals called **amino acids**. These are essential for a balanced diet. Some amino acids we can make for ourselves, others are obtained from the foods that we eat.

There are two types of protein; both types provide the remaining amino acids that the body needs.

- Animal protein – from products such as meat, fish, eggs, milk and cheese.
- Vegetable protein – from plant products such as peas, beans, lentils and nuts. They are a very good source of protein for vegetarians. A mixed vegetable diet is needed to provide all the essential amino acids.

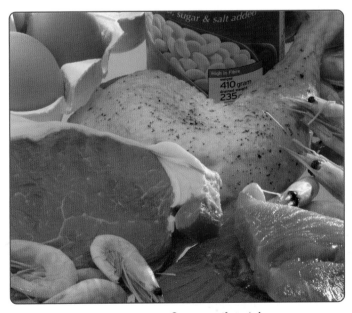

Sources of protein

 Worksheet 25 – Positive and negative factors

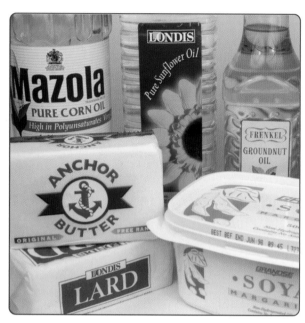

Sources of fat

Word check

cholesterol – fatty substance needed by the body and carried in the blood.

Word check

kilojoule – unit of energy.
Calorie – unit of energy.

Fats

Fats are very good for providing the body with energy and are found in both animal and vegetable products. There are two main types of fat:

- saturated fats
- unsaturated fats.

Saturated fats

These are found in both animal and vegetable products. Products like meat, milk and eggs are high in saturated fats. Saturated fats are also found in some vegetable products like coconut oil.

Saturated fats are important to our body but we do have to limit the amount we eat. This because too much saturated fat can give us high levels of **cholesterol** in our blood, which can increase our risk of heart disease. High levels of cholesterol cause a build up of fatty deposits in the arteries. This narrows the arteries and can lead to heart attacks.

Unsaturated fats

These are found in vegetable products and some fish. Vegetable oils, sunflower oil, olive oil, herring and cod liver oil are valuable sources of unsaturated fat. These fats do not raise our blood cholesterol.

Carbohydrate

Carbohydrates provide the body with energy, but their energy value is not as high as that in fat. Most of our carbohydrates come from sugars and starches. Foods such as biscuits, chocolate, cakes, honey and jams are high in carbohydrate. A second source of carbohydrates is foods such as pasta, rice and potatoes. These also provide a high energy source. In both fat and carbohydrate we can measure this energy in units known as **kilojoules** or **Calories**. These are the same Calories that people count in their diets.

11 Make a list of what you had to eat yesterday. What dietary components did it contain? Look back at page 103 to see the seven essential components.

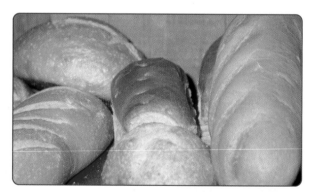

Bread is a good source of carbohydrate

Vitamins

Vitamins are found in most of the food that we eat. The main vitamins are listed in the table below. Their main function is to regulate the chemical processes that take place in our body. See too, the Daily recommended vitamin intake table in the Appendix (page 265).

Appendix 1, see page 265

Vitamin	What it does	Found in	Effect if absent
Vitamin A	Necessary for new cells to grow and to fight infection. Gives healthy skin, blood, strong bones, healthy teeth, kidneys, bladder; helps good eyesight.	Fish liver oils, liver, dairy foods, carrots, peaches, tomatoes, sweet potatoes, apricots, green and yellow fruit and vegetables	Unable to see in the dark; skin problems.
B-Complex	The B-Complex vitamins help in energy production. They are important for the way the nervous system works; healthy hair, skin, eyes, liver, mouth, and muscle tone and blood production.	Brewer's yeast, liver, wholegrain cereals	Problems in the nervous system; muscle weakness and skin problems; beri-beri; anaemia; mouth ulcers and nerve damage.
Vitamin C	Helps in the production of red blood cells and in healing; fights bacterial infections; helps to combat the effects of stress.	Citrus fruits and berries, green vegetables, onions, tomatoes, rose hip syrup, green peppers	Scurvy; cuts and wounds are slow to heal; infections are more likely to occur.
Vitamin D	Promotes strong bones and teeth; helps in prevention of rickets; protects against muscle weakness; helps regulate the heart and contributes to good health.	Fish, fish liver oil, egg yolks, milk, dairy products	Rickets in children; weak bones and muscles.
Vitamin E	Helps muscles use oxygen; improves circulation; helps normal clotting and healing; extends life of red blood cells; makes skin soft; keeps eyes healthy.	Most vegetables, raw seeds and nuts, eggs, leafy vegetables, beef, liver, milk, eggs, butter, rice, wholemeal bread	Prevents wound healing and normal functioning of the nervous system.
Vitamin K	Aids blood clotting; essential for normal liver function; helps calcium to be absorbed.	Leafy green vegetables, milk, yogurt, egg yolks, polyunsaturated oils, fish liver oils	Bruising

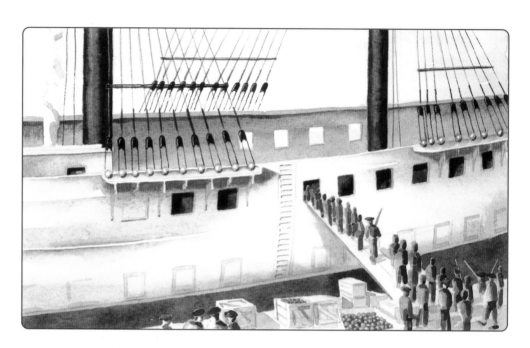

Oranges are a good source of vitamin C

We need to obtain small amounts of vitamins from our food. If any vitamins are absent from our diet their deficiency can cause health problems. In the 17th and 18th centuries, English sailors constantly suffered from a disease called scurvy. Scurvy is caused by a deficiency in Vitamin C, which gave the sailors skin problems, bleeding gums and caused their teeth to fall out. It was eventually stopped when they found that Spanish sailors did not have this problem because they ate oranges as part of their diet on board ship.

12 List FIVE foods that contain vitamin C.

Minerals

Minerals are found in most of the foods that we eat. Some foods contain larger amounts of **minerals** than others. They are essential in maintaining our body function. Certain minerals, such as calcium, are important in bone growth and repair. The mineral table opposite shows the main minerals that we need. It also shows what they do and the foods that are rich in them. The body uses many different minerals so the table presents the most important ones. See too, the daily recommended mineral intake in the Appendix (page 265).

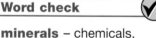

Word check

minerals – chemicals, some of which are needed as nutrients in our diet.

Appendix 2, see page 265

Nutrient	Babies	Children	Men 19–65	Men over 65	Women 19–55	Women over 55
Calcium (mg)	525	450	800	800	800	1000
Iodine (mg)			150	150	120	120
Iron (mg)	1.7	6.1	7	7	12.6	5.7

Mineral	Use	Found in
Calcium	Builds strong bones and teeth; muscle growth; aids blood clotting and heart rhythm; transmission of nerve impulses; prevents bone loss associated with osteoporosis.	Milk and milk products, yogurt, cheese, whole grains, green vegetables, sardines, salmon, soya beans, peanuts
Chromium	Helps bring protein to where it's needed; necessary for energy production and the proper use of cholesterol, fats and proteins.	Meats, brewer's yeast, unsaturated fats, vegetable oil, liver, wholegrain cereal, chicken, shellfish
Iron	Required for the production of red blood cells; increases resistance to disease; increases energy production.	Lean meats, brewer's yeast, liver, eggs, wholegrain bread and cereals, vegetables, heart, kidney beans, peas, fish, poultry, prunes, prune juice, oysters
Magnesium	Functioning of nerves and muscles; maintenance of bones; helps protect the arteries; helps the body form its bones and proteins; aids blood clotting and creation of new cells.	Peas, dark green vegetables, nuts, wholegrain foods, dry beans, soya products
Manganese	Necessary for normal skeletal development; helps maintain sex hormone production; nourishes the nerves and brain.	Egg yolks, sunflower seeds, wheatgerm, wholegrain cereals, flour, dried peas, brewer's yeast
Phosphorous	Maintenance, repair of cells and energy production; necessary for skeletal growth and tooth development.	Fish, whole grains, meat, seeds, nuts
Potassium	Required for muscles, nerves and heart; aids maintenance of mineral balance of blood as well as a stable blood pressure; helps to regulate the body's water balance.	Whole grains, green leafy vegetables, sunflower seeds, potatoes (preferably unpeeled), bananas, lean meat, avocados, apricots, orange juice, dried fruits, cooked dried beans, peas
Selenium	A required trace mineral, selenium supports the body's immune system, helps the body produce antibodies and helps the heart stay healthy.	Broccoli, bran, onions, tomatoes, tuna, wheatgerm, swordfish, salmon, cracked wheat bread, selenium-rich yeast, sunflower seeds, oysters
Zinc	Required for healing and development of new cells; helps enzymes in digestion and metabolism; needed for general growth, reproductive organs, normal functioning of prostate gland. Zinc is thought to help the body repair wounds, synthesise protein, preserve vision and boost the immune system.	Bonemeal, fish, brewer's yeast, beans, nuts, seeds, wheatgerm, meat, liver, oysters, poultry, organ meats, wholegrain bread and cereals, pumpkin seeds

Water

Water is the most important part of our diet. We can go without food for weeks and still survive. However, without drinking water we will die in a matter of days. All our body processes take place in water. It helps us digest our food and dispose of our waste products. We should all realise the great value of water.

How much water do we need?

A good rule to follow is to drink half your weight in fluid ounces of water every day.

So, if you weigh 98 pounds you would benefit by drinking 49 fluid ounces of water each day. This is almost two and a half pints.

If you are using metric measurements then you can divide your weight in kilograms by 33. This gives you the amount of water needed in litres.

So, 44.5kg (98lbs) divided by 33 is 1.35 litres of water daily.

These methods are approximate guides.

Water is found in fruit juices, teas, sparkling water and other fizzy drinks. Drinking pure water allows your body to wash out **toxins** without putting stress on your digestive system. Drinking water is one of the single most important tasks we do daily in order to live a long and healthy life.

13 How much water should you drink a day?

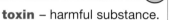
Word check ✓

toxin – harmful substance.

Word check ✓

constipation – inability to have a bowel movement.

Fibre

Fibre in our diet adds bulk to the food that we eat. This helps our digestive system to move the food through the bowel (large intestine).

We find fibre in a variety of different foods, such as:

- bran
- rice
- whole grain cereals
- wholemeal bread
- fruit
- vegetables (peas, beans, greens).

Without fibre in our diet we may suffer from poor digestion of our food, which can also lead to **constipation**.

14 Where does your daily fibre come from?

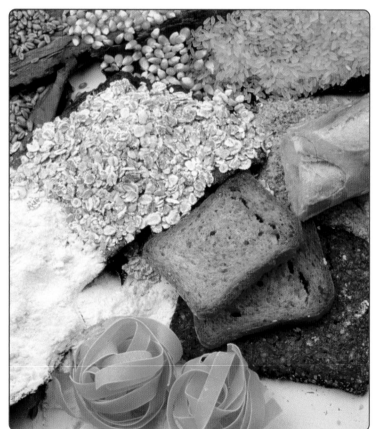

Sources of fibre

Eating a healthy balanced diet

A healthy diet contains all the **nutrients** needed by the body. Nutritionists have worked out a rough guide to show what a healthy diet should include. This is what they recommend.

> **Word check** ✓
>
> **nutrient** – valuable part of our food.

Fruit and vegetables

Scientific studies have shown that if we eat a lot of fruit and vegetables we are usually healthier. We may have a lower risk of developing heart disease and some cancers. For this reason, it is recommended that we eat at least five portions of fruit and vegetables every day. It does not matter whether they are fresh, tinned, frozen, cooked, juiced or dried.

But what does a portion look like?

- One medium-sized fruit, for example, an apple, peach, banana or orange.
- One slice of a large fruit, such as melon, mango or pineapple.
- A few handfuls of grapes, or berry fruits.
- A small handful of dried fruit.
- A glass (100ml) of fruit or vegetable juice.
- A small tin (200g) of fruit.
- A side salad.
- A serving (100g) of vegetables, for example frozen or tinned peas, boiled carrots or stir-fried vegetables.
- The vegetables served in a portion of vegetable curry, lasagne, stir fry or casserole.

How does this translate into everyday eating?

- Glass of fruit juice for breakfast (one portion).
- Small pack of dried apricots for mid-morning snack (instead of that chocolate bar or bag of crisps) (one portion).
- Side salad with lunch (one portion).
- Peas, beans or carrots, served with main meal (one portion).
- Fruit for dessert (one portion).

15 How many portions of fruit and vegetables do you need each day?

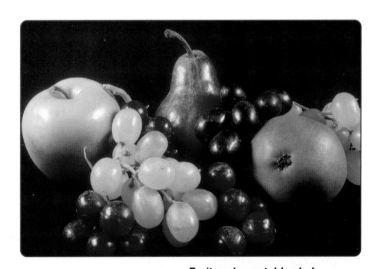

Fruit and vegetables help to protect us from infection

Word check

bulk – the biggest part.

Carbohydrate

It is recommended that bread, cereals, pasta and potatoes make up the **bulk** of our diet. This should be roughly 50%. This is not usually difficult as most of our meals contain at least one of these.

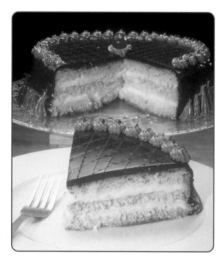

We should eat less of this

Sugary foods

The suggestion for sugary foods is that we eat less. If you would like to cut down on sugary foods, snack on fresh or dried fruit rather than biscuits and chocolate.

Protein

Nutritionists recommend that protein makes up 10–15% of our diet. They suggest that adult men eat 55.5g of protein every day, and adult women eat 45g every day. Eating a moderate amount of protein in one or two meals every day should give us all the protein we need. We all need to eat the correct amount of protein daily because our bodies cannot store protein. We cannot stock up on it by bingeing. Simply eating a variety of foods every day is all you need to do.

Fats

Word check

intake – what is taken in.
supplement – something extra, to add to.

Government targets recommend that fat makes up no more than 35% of our diet. No more than 10% of this fat should be saturated fat. For the average woman, this means about 76g of fat per day and, for a man, this means roughly 100g of fat per day.

In reality though, most of us have higher fat **intakes** than this. The secret is not to have too much of one thing. We all need fat in our diet, the idea is not to overdo it.

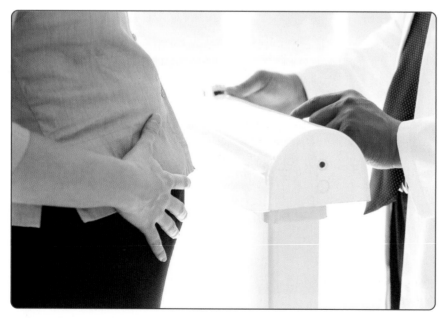

Vitamins and minerals

Everyone needs vitamins and minerals in their daily diet. Sometimes people need to **supplement** their diet. Pregnant mothers are a good example as they are effectively eating to provide for their baby as well. They are therefore often given vitamin and mineral supplements in tablet form. Just like the food we eat there is a recommended daily intake for vitamins and minerals so we can work out what we require. (See the Mineral and Vitamin charts in the Appendix, page 265.)

A pregnant mother needs to make sure she has a balanced diet

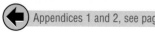

Appendices 1 and 2, see page 265
 16 Why is it important to have a balanced diet?

Calories and calories, Kilojoules and joules

So where do calories and joules fit into our diet? The calorie and joule are units used to measure the amount of energy that the body uses. We can use these terms for measuring energy values of food. We also use them to measure the energy we burn off in exercise.

The calorie (with a small 'c') is 1/1000th of a Calorie (with a capital 'C') that you see on food packets. Therefore the Calorie is the one commonly used for measurements of energy.

- 1 calorie = 4.2 joules
- 1000 calories = 1kilocal or 1 Calorie (1 Cal)
- 1 kilocalorie = 4.2 kilojoules

This means that we can work in Calories but the modern internationally agreed system of measurement (SI) usually uses kilojoules. You will see all of these on food and drink packaging.

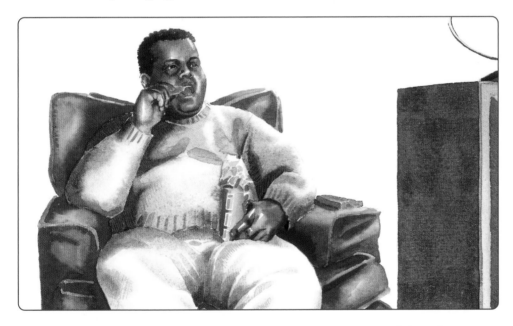

Too little activity and too much food can make us put on weight

On average we use between 500 and 700 Calories (2100–2940 kilojoules) every day just to stay alive. While we are sitting watching the television and resting we do not use much energy. At rest the body burns about 12 Calories of energy for every pound of our weight (approximately 112 kilojoules per kilogram). So let us see how many Calories/kilojoules you burn at rest if you weigh 7 stone (98lbs or 45kg).

Example:

12 (Calories) x 98 (lbs) = 1176 Calories.

112 (kilojoules) x 45 (kg) = 5040 kilojoules

That means that someone who weighs 7 stone uses approximately 1176 Calories or 5040 kilojoules in one day at rest.

17 How many Calories do you need each day if you weigh 67kg?

Appendix 3, see page 265

 Appendix 4, see page 266

By using this simple formula we can see if someone's diet is correct. This is because all foods have a calorie value. Look at the Calorie counter in the Appendix (page 266) and the energy values given in Appendix 3 (page 265).

Food	Measure	Calories
Milk (full cream)	1 cup	167
Milk (skimmed)	1 cup	88
Milk (soya)	1 cup	160
Yogurt (natural)	200g	160

Calorie counter

 Appendix 6, see page 269

This will help you create healthy diets. It will also help to make sure that you are eating the right foods. Some examples of healthy diet plans can be found in the Appendix (page 269).

Finding out about diet   ACTIVITY

A1 Keep a diary of everything that you eat and drink in a week. Calculate the following:

- How many portions of fruit and vegetables have you eaten?

- How many bags of crisps or similar snacks have you eaten?

- How many Calories were in the crisps? The packet will tell you how many Calories are in a bag.

- Work out a menu for an evening meal for yourself. Show how it is well balanced.

A2 Copy and complete the sentences using suitable words.

Protein helps to _____, _____ and _____. Protein foods can be found in _____, _____ and _____.

There are _____ main types of protein.

A3 Miranda, aged 16, has the following for her evening meal: beefburger, chips, tomato and chocolate.

- Show the main nutrients that are in the meal and explain how Miranda could make the meal well balanced.

- Plan a meal for Miranda that is well balanced. Explain why it is well balanced.

Exercise

Now we know what to eat, what do we need to know about exercise? Firstly, we all need exercise; it is no good saying, 'I've been very busy, I've had enough exercise for one day'. If we fail to exercise properly on a regular basis we may suffer from one or more of these problems:

- coronary heart disease
- **cardio-vascular** problems
- **obesity**
- **osteoporosis**
- muscle and joint problems.

Exercise helps to keep us fit. It strengthens our body, helps to control our weight and burns off extra energy. It has a great many other health benefits too, because it:

- improves our **circulation**
- helps our heart work more efficiently
- improves the strength in our muscles
- improves our **stamina**
- reduces the risk of heart attack
- improves our **mobility**
- helps in building up our **immunity**.

If we take no exercise we may be putting our health at risk, and exercise has other positive effects on our well-being. It has many **psychological** effects, for example:

- builds confidence
- helps relieve stress
- improves self-esteem
- gives a general feeling of well-being
- it is a great way to socialise.

Word check

cardio-vascular – relating to heart and blood vessels.
obesity – very overweight.
osteoporosis – condition related to bones caused by deficiency of calcium.

Word check

circulation – movement of blood around the body.
stamina – ability to keep going.
mobility – ability to move.

Word check

immunity – resistance to a disease.
psychological – relating to the mind.

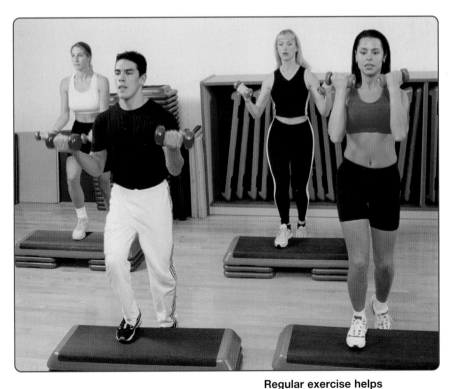

Regular exercise helps us to keep fit

Exercise changes our body's composition. It increases the amount of muscle we have and reduces our fat levels. Babies, from the moment that they are born, begin to exercise their muscles. Children exercise in all their activities and sport is a major part of growing up for most people. It protects our physical as well as our emotional well-being. It also helps protect us against diseases in later life such as osteoporosis.

18 Why is exercise important?

Aerobic exercise

Aerobic exercises include walking, jogging and swimming. They involve muscles moving through their full range over set time periods (15–20 minutes). These activities are additional to our normal daily routine. During the activities the heart and breathing rates increase. This type of exercise is used to improve cardio-vascular fitness. It increases blood flow to the muscles and benefits the whole body.

Aerobic exercises should be planned to increase the heart rate to 70% of its maximum. The maximum rate is 220 beats per minute (bpm), minus the person's age. This provides a safety barrier to help reduce any danger from excessive exercise.

Example:

The maximum heart rate for a 45 year-old is:

220 − 45 = 175

70% of 175 = 123

Therefore, a fit 45 year-old should be able to exercise safely at 123bpm.

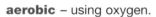

Word check

aerobic – using oxygen.

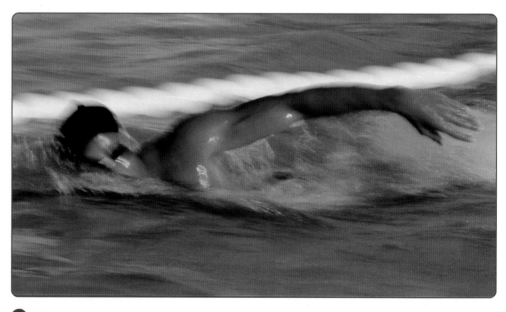

Swimming is one type of aerobic exercise

19 What should your maximum heart rate be when you are exercising if you are 19 years old?

Aerobic exercise is the most commonly used method of increasing and maintaining fitness. It must be remembered that exercising above the safe rate can be dangerous.

Anaerobic exercise

Anaerobic exercise is the body builders' method of building muscle. It involves high intensity activity, aimed at developing the muscles. It is only carried on for short periods of time.

Weightlifting is a good example of an anaerobic exercise. Anaerobic activities increase the amount of muscle and strength. Benefits to the heart and the lungs are limited by using this method.

20 What is the difference between aerobic and anaerobic?

Word check ✓

anaerobic – not using oxygen.

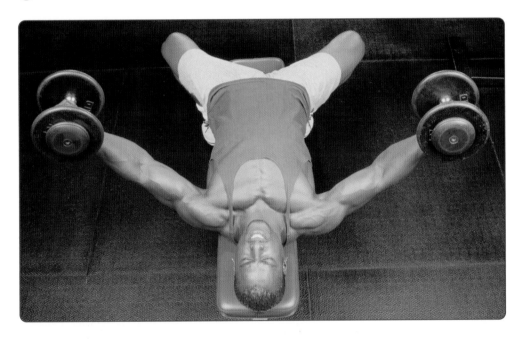

An example of an anaerobic exercise

Exercising safely

When starting exercise, beginners ideally should be supervised. They should be made aware of the dangers of over exercising, especially the strain that they can put on their heart and circulation. Making muscles work to the point of exhaustion is dangerous. If a person's health and heart are poor this can bring on a collapse or a heart attack. Exercise should always be moderate and not excessive. It should also be regular. This allows the body to build up stamina and lessens the risk of injury.

Which are the best exercises?

Just as certain foods are better for us than others, so are certain exercises. Exercise should start off at an easy pace. Eventually we should be doing 30 minutes' exercise at least three times a week. Remember exercise should not make you exceed 70% of your maximum heart rate. Taking part in exercise regularly can develop your interest in the activity as you enjoy it. Look at the Exercise table on the next page. This shows the amount of Calories used by carrying out each activity for 30 minutes.

This table can be used to help work out exercises for different people. It includes exercises for all ages and abilities.

21 Why is safety important when exercising?

**Exercise table for a person weighing 160 pounds
(exercising for 30 minutes)**

Activity	Calories used
aerobics	214
basketball	286
boating	89
bowling	107
canoeing	143
cooking	89
cycling (leisurely)	214
dancing	161
driving	71
fishing	143
football	286
gardening	179
golf	161
hiking	214
horse-riding	143
house cleaning	89
jogging	250
mountain biking	125
playing guitar	107
playing piano	89
squash	358
rock climbing	393
running (5mph)	286
cross-country	322
running on the spot	286
running upstairs	537
shopping	82
watching TV	35
skiing	250
sleeping	32
football	250
exercise bike	214
reading	64
swimming	286
talking on the phone	35
tennis	250
volleyball	107
walking (4mph)	125
weightlifting	107
writing	35
yoga	143

Whether you are young or old, fit, unfit or disabled, you can always find some form of exercise to suit your age or condition. Being fit is becoming very fashionable, which fits in nicely with the government's health plans. The final point to remember is:

– to lose one kilogram in weight you have to burn off 8000 Calories or 33 600 kilojoules (3500 Calories per pound in weight).

Learning about exercise ACTIVITY

A1 Carry out some research to find out TWO other types of aerobic and TWO other types of anaerobic exercises.

A2 Keep a diary of how much exercise you do during one week. How much did you do? Draw some conclusions about the amount of exercise you have done and how this contributes to your health status.

A3 Create a plan of regular exercise for yourself or for a friend for one week. Make sure the exercises can be done safely. Explain how the exercises will help to improve or maintain fitness.

A4 Carry out the Harvard step test either on yourself or the friend you have chosen (see worksheet 28). Record your findings.

A5 Draw some conclusions about your own or your friend's health status. How would you use this information when drawing up a health plan?

A6 If someone takes regular exercise and becomes fit, how do you think the improvements will affect their physical, intellectual, emotional and social health and well-being?

Sleep

Sleep is an essential part of our daily routine. The amount we need varies with our age. It is well known that babies, toddlers, pregnant mothers and some older people need to rest during the day. Sleep helps to refresh the body and restore our energy reserves. While we are asleep the body has the opportunity to carry out repairs to our systems.

As we grow we develop sleep patterns that change with age. A newborn baby will normally only sleep for a few hours at any one time. By three months they may sleep right through the night. When children reach five years of age they have usually given up the daytime nap. As we get older the amount of sleep we take depends on our individual need. Adults sleep between four and ten hours a day. Many older people find that they begin to need less sleep.

A good night's sleep is very important. If you do not get enough sleep everything you do is affected. You become tired, irritable and confused; you make mistakes; your hearing and vision may become impaired. This is why drivers are told, 'tiredness kills'.

22 Why is sleep important?

Supportive relationships and good health

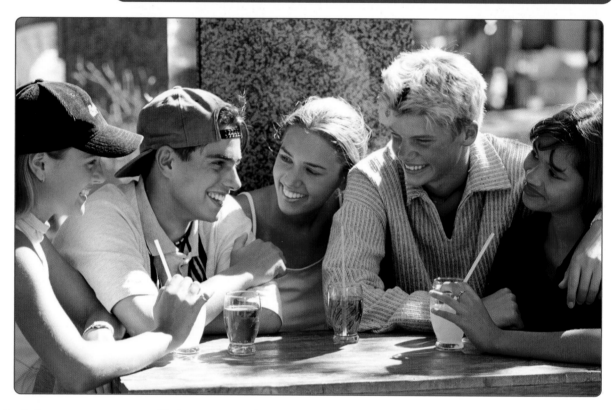

Sharing and caring helps us to feel good about ourselves.

Word check

gregarious – enjoy the company of others.

Word check

immune system – body's system to protect against disease.

Generally humans tend to be **gregarious**. This means that we like mixing with other people. Our health and well-being can be affected by the relationships that we make. Having supportive relationships at home makes us feel secure and happy – major factors in feeling good. When we feel good we have pride in ourselves. We look after ourselves and this helps us remain healthy.

If we are not sharing time with others and if our relationships are not giving us support our self-esteem can become very low. We may end up not liking ourselves or other people. In extreme cases we may feel suicidal. Supportive relationships are, therefore, very important. They can lift our self-esteem and make us feel positive about ourselves. We need this feeling of good 'self-concept' to stay healthy. The mind is a powerful force and people act according to how they feel about themselves. If we wake up in the morning and everything around us is good, we tend to feel good all day. If we wake up and think our relationships are not working, we are more likely to have a bad day. We all have days when we do not feel very good about ourselves. If this lasts for a long period of time we could become depressed. Eventually our health will be affected. This can lead to the **immune system** also being affected. We then become more prone to illness.

23 What does it mean to be gregarious?

How leisure activities can help health and well-being

Leisure and recreational activities play a vital role in keeping us healthy. Many of the leisure activities we participate in involve us in meeting others. This can provide a great boost to our well-being. We can become part of a team, join in with group activities or even just be with one other person in our leisure activities. Examples of leisure activities are chess, drama clubs, martial arts, pottery, learning a new language or skill. Taking part in activities is a basic part of community and family life.

24 Why do we need to socialise with other people?

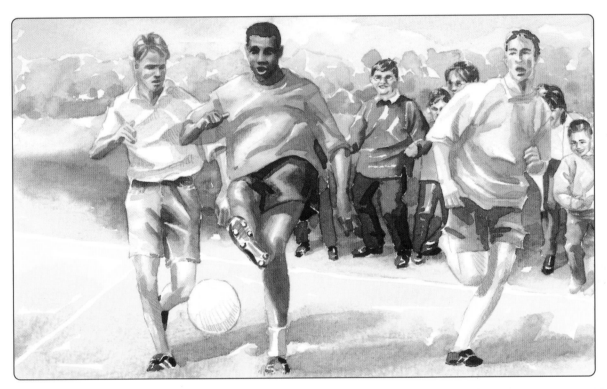

Leisure activities can
bring people together

Work, money and social class

Our work and the money that we earn can be linked to health and well-being because it influences what we are able to do. If we work we earn money. If we have money we can buy the things we need and want. Money also allows us to socialise, as we can go out to the cinema or to a club, for example.

At work we may get a lot of social enjoyment from our colleagues. This can have a very positive effect on our health and well-being. Working gives our lives structure, a framework that we build everything else around. If we are working we are likely to have more confidence and self-respect. Our status at work can give us a psychological boost and make us feel important.

Unemployment can have a negative effect on people and their families. If someone is unemployed for any length of time they could suffer from:

- depression
- stress
- financial insecurity (money problems)
- anxiety
- lack of confidence
- low self-esteem
- insomnia (inability to sleep)
- worry.

Single parents or the main wage earner often feel under a lot of pressure to work and earn an income. When people start suffering from any of the conditions given above, then work can be more difficult to obtain and this may in turn affect our health. The ability to work and to earn puts us in control. Knowing that we are in control of our lives helps us to remain healthy.

25 How does being unemployed affect our self-esteem?

Education as a contributor to health and well-being

Education plays an important part in health and well-being. The better our education, the more choices are open to us. A good all-round education appears to have a real impact on our lives.

Our willingness to learn makes us **inquisitive** and this helps us to make the best choices; such as which job we would like or whether to go to university or which parts of the world we want to see. Life is full of choices and to make the best decisions we need to use our intellect to think through situations carefully. Knowledge also allows us to manage risks better.

Word check ✓

inquisitive – curious, eager to learn.

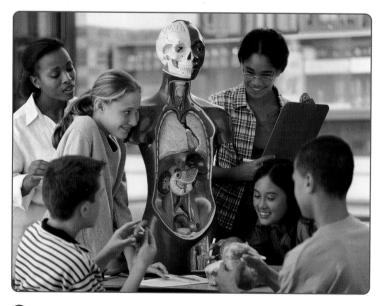

Learning can help to stimulate the mind

26 Why is health education important?

Health monitoring and disease prevention

Preventing disease is a way of helping us to stay healthy for longer. Some diseases are not always visible and can be difficult to detect. It is possible for a person to have a disease without being aware of it. Diseases like tuberculosis may not show any symptoms for up to six months. For this reason many different ways of detection and prevention have been developed.

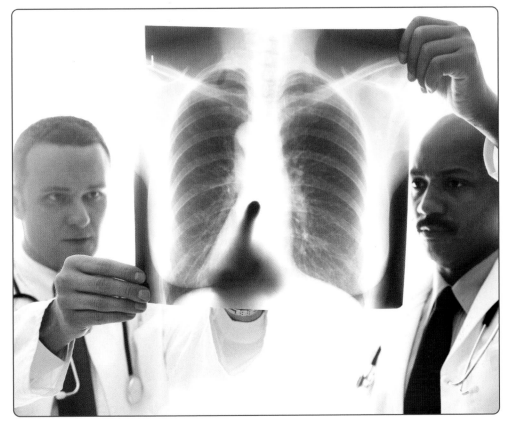

An X-ray can show disease

Health care professionals use tests like chest X-rays and blood tests to help detect illness and disease. These show changes in the person caused by the disease. A chest X-ray provides a picture of any infection in the lungs. A blood test may show chemical changes in the body. Where these tests are done on a large scale they are known as screening programmes. Screening allows doctors to examine many people and to select those that need treatment because disease has been found.

Screening can include:

- childhood blood tests
- **cervical smear** tests
- chest X-rays
- **breast screening**.

These tests are all done to find out if a problem exists.

27 Why do we need to test people for diseases?

Word check

cervical smear – testing the neck of the uterus for signs of cancer.

Word check

breast screening – checking the breasts for signs of cancer.

Preventing disease

You may have heard the phrase 'prevention is better than cure'.

Some diseases are so dangerous that we have had to find methods of preventing them occurring. **Vaccination** programmes have been running in the UK for over 50 years. People who have a high risk of catching certain illnesses, can have medical help to prevent this happening. The vaccine is usually given by injection.

> **Word check** ✓
>
> **vaccination** – using a substance to prevent disease.

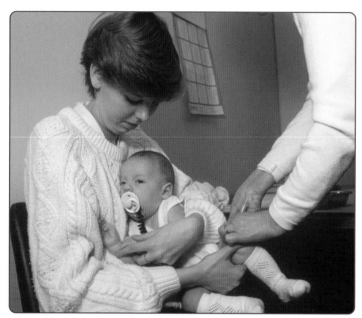

Vaccination helps prevent diseases

In the past a killer disease called smallpox was totally eliminated because people all over the world were vaccinated against it. More recently, vaccinations to prevent measles, mumps and rubella (MMR) and influenza (flu) have become available. These have been introduced because these diseases can kill vulnerable people, such as children and older adults.

28 Why do we vaccinate small children?

Risk management

How can risk management promote good health? Personal safety is an important aspect of our lives. This applies equally at home, in a public place or at work. Staying safe is our responsibility. Accidents are responsible for 10 000 deaths each year in England. A large number of people are disabled as a result of accidents.

Many accidents in the home could be avoided. Children are most at risk, as are older adults. Dangerous items such as sharp knives, scissors, household chemicals and kettles with boiling water should be kept out of children's reach. For the safety of older adults we need to make sure that lighting is adequate, that carpets are not loose so that they do not trip over and that there are no obstacles on the stairs. We need to know how to reduce **hazards**.

> **Word check** ✓
>
> **hazard** – a danger.

Risk management is more likely to be applied in public places such as hospitals, residential homes and playgroups, and in places of work.

Employers are responsible for the health and safety of their employees and for those in their care. A risk assessment would be carried out to find out what the risks are. Methods for reducing the risks would then be put in place. For example, to reduce risk from fire, smoke detectors and fire alarms can be installed and checks made to make sure fire exits are not blocked.

We have a responsibility not to put ourselves or others at risk.

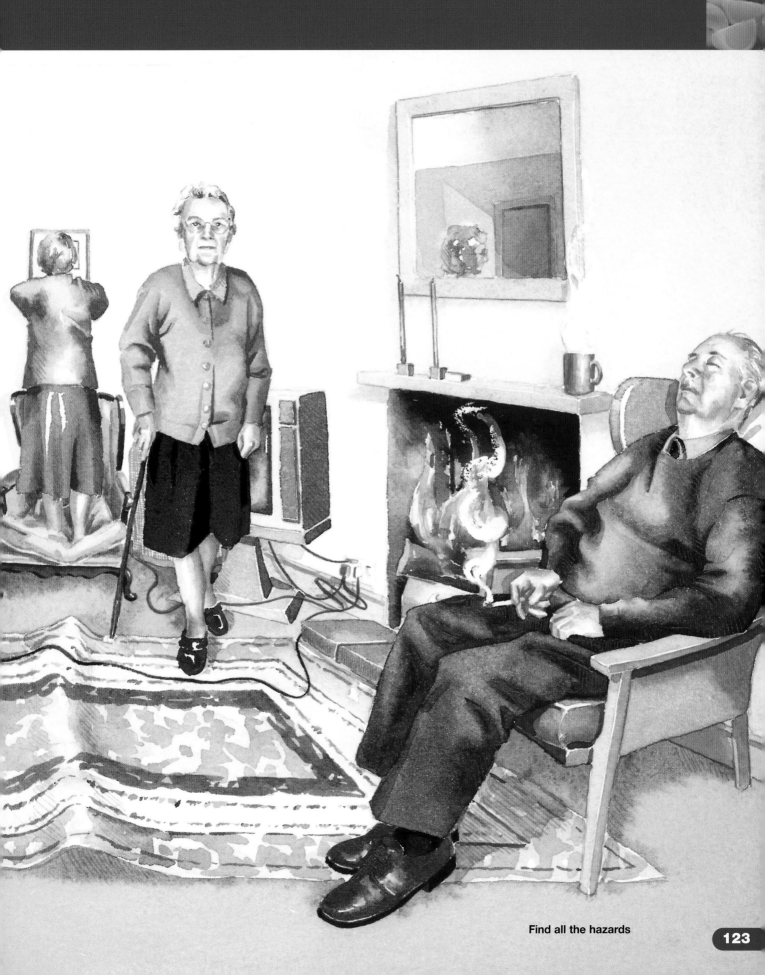

Find all the hazards

Reducing the risks

ACTIVITY

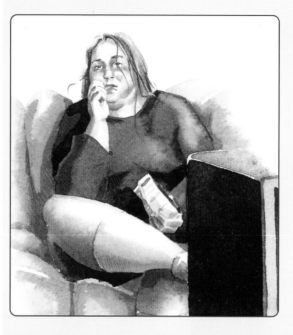

Marlene has very low self-esteem

Marlene is 20. She has left school and is unable to get work.

She spends most of her time watching TV but occasionally visits her friend Sandra for a chat. Marlene eats a lot of chocolate and crisps and has become very overweight. She does not like going out any more because she is so fat. She often wakes up with a start in the middle of the night and then she cannot get back to sleep.

A1 Identify the factors that are negatively affecting Marlene's health and well-being.

A2 Draw up a plan for three days to help Marlene improve her physical, intellectual, emotional and social well-being.

  • Explain why the plan will work for Marlene.

Patrina is expecting her first child.

A3 What tests could Patrina have to find out if her unborn child is healthy?

A4 Produce a leaflet or a handout to give Patrina information and advice about vaccinations available for young children.

A residential home wants to carry out a risk assessment of the residents' lounge.

A5 What advice would you give them to help them with this task?

A6 Draw up a check list that would help them conduct the risk assessment.

A7 Produce a leaflet or handout that could be used by someone to help them carry out a risk assessment of their kitchen.

Genetics and inherited diseases

We share some of our physical features with other people. The reason for this is we share similar genes. Long before anyone used the terms **gene** and **DNA**, it was well-known that physical characteristics could be passed down from parent to child.

> **Word check** ✓
>
> **DNA** – (deoxyribonucleic acid) your body blueprint found in the cells.

> **Word check** ✓
>
> **gene** – part of a chromosome that controls a particular characteristic, for example, eye colour.

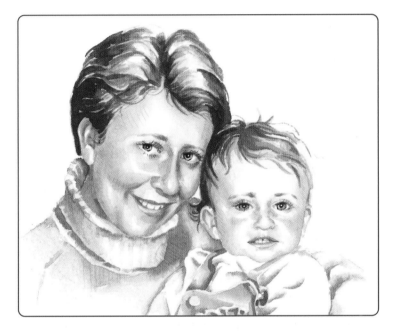

Hair colour is a characteristic often passed from parent to child

This means that diseases can also be passed down the family line by harmful or 'non-functioning' genes. If genes are harmful or if they do not function properly, then neither do our bodies. Almost every in-built strength or weakness we have is determined in part by our genes. Examples are the ability to run fast or short-sightedness. These can be passed down from our mother or father or from grandparents.

There are many physical problems and diseases that can be **inherited** genetically; these are some of the most common:

- heart conditions
- eye conditions (**glaucoma**, short and long sight)
- hypertension (high blood pressure)
- schizophrenia (personality disorder)
- **diabetes insipidus**
- haemophilia (inability of blood to clot)
- high cholesterol
- achondraplasia (dwarfism)
- cystic fibrosis
- Down's syndrome
- baldness (fortunately for women, mainly in men).

> **Word check** ✓
>
> **inherited** – genetic information passed from parent to children.

> **Word check** ✓
>
> **glaucoma** – eye disease that may cause blindness.
> **diabetes insipidus** – disease that stops the body properly using and regulating sugar.

So how are these problems passed on?

In the nucleus of almost every cell in our body we have a genetic code. This is a blueprint of how we are made up and how we look. This blueprint of information is carried on chromosomes in what are known as genes. By passing on these genes to our children they can inherit our characteristics.

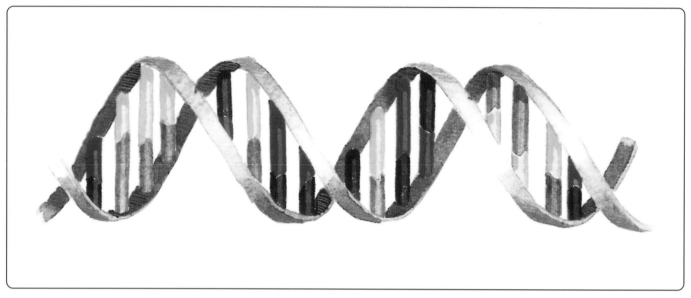

DNA double helix

We each have a set number of chromosomes. In body cells there are 46 chromosomes (23 pairs). In reproductive cells (egg and sperm cells) there are 23 chromosomes. This allows egg and sperm cells to join together on fertilization to give a new cell. The new cell has the correct number of chromosomes; half from each parent. The cell then divides to create a person with their own individual genetic make up, based on both their parents.

The sex chromosomes are called X and Y. If you are male then the pair will be made up of one X and one Y chromosome. If you are female then they will both be X chromosomes. All chromosomes carry genes that hold information about our make up.

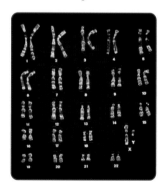

These chromosomes make us who we are

29 How many chromosome pairs are there in body cells?

30 Why do children often look like one of their parents?

Gene defects

There are four basic forms of gene defect that create inherited problems:

- dominant gene defects
- recessive gene defects
- X-linked recessive gene defects
- chromosomal defects.

Dominant gene defects

A person with a dominant gene defect only needs to have one defective gene to suffer from the defect. A parent with a dominant gene defect has a 50% chance of passing that defect on to their children. For example, if one parent suffers from dwarfism, then the child will have a 50% chance of suffering dwarfism too.

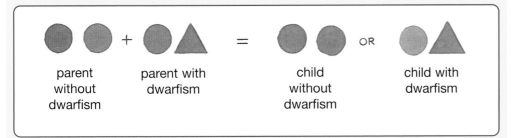

Dominant gene defects carry the highest risk

Recessive gene defects

A person with a recessive gene defect must have two defective genes in order to suffer from the defect. These defects are only inherited if the **carriers** of two recessive genes reproduce. If both parents carry the same recessive gene then there is a 25% chance that the child will inherit the problem. Cystic fibrosis is an example of a disease that is inherited this way. The diagram shows how children who do not have cystic fibrosis still have a high risk of being carriers of the gene.

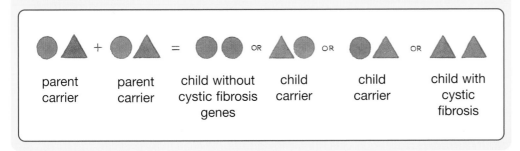

Recessive gene defects carry a lower risk

X-linked recessive gene defects

In these conditions the gene is only on the X chromosome. This usually leads to the abnormality occurring in males only. Women can be carriers of the defect and 50% of their sons may be affected. An example of this is haemophilia.

Chromosomal defects

These vary considerably because either the structure or the number of chromosomes can vary. Fetuses that have this type of defect often naturally abort. This is known as a **miscarriage**. 0.5% of babies born have some type of chromosomal abnormality. An example of this type of defect is that which causes Down's syndrome. Children with Down's syndrome have three of chromosome 21, instead of the normal two. This is known as a trisomy.

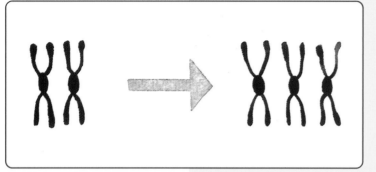

Down's syndrome: three chromosomes instead of two

Word check

miscarriage – natural abortion, loss of a fetus.

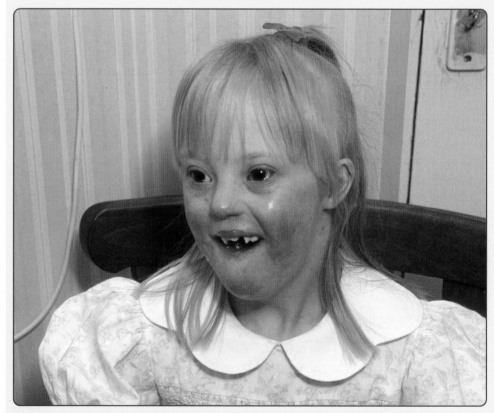

Down's syndrome is a result of chromosomal abnormality

How external influences affect us

Sometimes genetic make up can be influenced by the environment in which we live and work. Certain chemicals are known to be **carcinogens** and can cause us to develop cancer if we come into contact with them. Phenol and benzene are two particularly dangerous chemicals. They are usually only found in industrial processes and are used under strictly controlled conditions.

Word check

carcinogen – substance that can cause cancer.

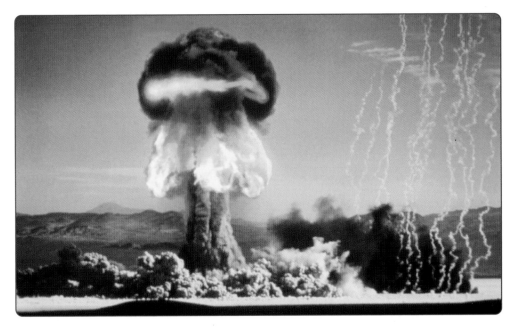

Environmental pollution

Possibly the greatest danger that we can be exposed to is nuclear radiation. In the normal course of our lives we all come into contact with natural radiation. It comes from the sun and is found in the ground beneath us. Nuclear accidents can happen. The last one of these was at Chernobyl in what was then the Soviet Union. Here a nuclear reactor in a power station exploded. This sprayed huge amounts of radioactive particles known as **fallout** into the atmosphere. The damage this caused to people's genetic structure created many extra cases of cancer and birth defects.

Word check

fallout – small radioactive particles that exist in the air after a nuclear explosion.

31 Why is radiation dangerous?

Many genetic defects can now be predicted by chemical tests or studying family history. These tests are supported by counselling. This is because of the psychological effect that a negative result can have on the parents.

Risks from genetically inherited diseases   ACTIVITY

A1 Carry out some research to find out about TWO different types of tests that can be used to discover whether an unborn child has a genetic condition or disease.

A2 Explain how cystic fibrosis is passed on.

A3 Explain how a dominant gene can affect the appearance of a child.

Substance misuse

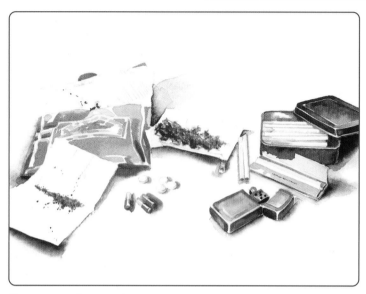

Drugs come in many forms

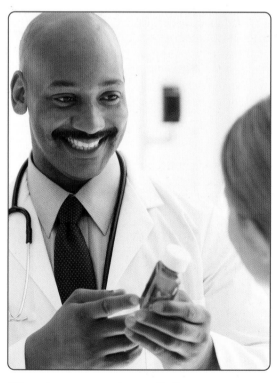

**When drugs are used correctly they can
help maintain health and well-being**

It is likely that you have already seen quite a lot of anti-drugs literature. You may have been told on many occasions by your teachers and parents that drugs are bad news. Some people take drugs as part of their 'medication'. The problem is not necessarily the drugs themselves but the attitude of the person that takes them. Anything taken in large amounts will cause the body to react to the substance.

The dictionary describes drugs as substances that are:

- used in medicine

- used as a stimulant

- used as a narcotic
  (causing sleep or drowsiness).

Drugs affect the body's chemistry. Our body chemistry is finely balanced to assist in the control of our bodily functions. Even the smallest changes can have a major effect on how we function.

To the doctor, drugs are one of the most valuable weapons in the fight against disease and illness. To obtain many of them we require a **prescription**. This is because if they are not given correctly some can be dangerous, if not fatal.

The correct amounts of prescribed drugs can be beneficial to the patient's health. In some circumstances prescribed drugs can have a negative effect. For example, taking certain drugs can lead to addiction.

Other types of drug can be obtained without a prescription because they have less risk. For, example, many painkillers can be bought over the counter in pharmacies and other shops. Care must be taken not to take more than the stated dose. These, too, can be harmful if taken in excess.

32 Why do we need prescriptions for certain drugs?

Let us look at two examples of use and abuse of drugs.

- A painkilling drug taken for a headache – taken as the packet says – is very effective at relieving the symptoms of a cold, headache or other minor pains. Taken to excess or overdose, it will cause liver failure and this can be fatal.

- A heart attack victim will be given various drugs when they reach the coronary care ward. Having a heart attack is extremely painful and requires very strong painkillers. In the hands of the doctor this has the effect of taking the pain of the attack away.

Many drugs can only be obtained on prescription. Some of the drugs are so strong that they are listed as **controlled drugs**. These drugs usually have powerful addictive properties. Doctors are always particularly careful when prescribing these drugs.

Word check

controlled drugs – drugs that are limited by law.

Word check

consequences – the effects of our actions.

Illegal drugs

Heroin is a form of drug. We all know that this drug wrecks lives and kills people.

What happens when a person's use of a chemical becomes uncontrolled, or it seems to control them? Even when there are serious **consequences** to their use of drugs, users may not want to stop. If and when they do decide to give up, they may find that it is harder than they thought.

This level of **dependency** on drugs is known as addiction. Taken over long periods of time, certain drugs make a person physically and psychologically dependent. Addicts who try to stop taking them experience very unpleasant side effects known as 'withdrawal symptoms'. These symptoms can range from bouts of depression to uncontrollable fits and convulsions. Amongst drug-users this is often given the slang term, **cold turkey**.

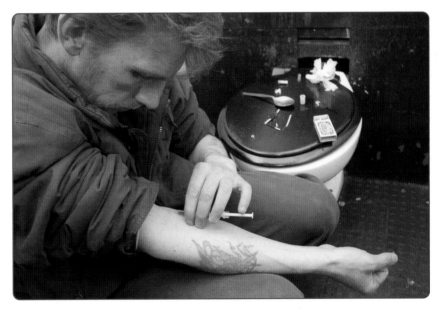

Used wrongly, heroin can kill

The Misuse of Drugs Act 1971 bans the non-medical use of controlled drugs. It makes the sale or possession of these drugs with the intention to supply, a serious criminal offence. Under new government law reforms offenders will serve lengthy prison sentences.

There are a great many illegal drugs now available to addicts and users – often manufactured in poor and dangerous conditions. This means that they may be mixed with other toxic substances and this forms an extra risk. Illegal drugs can be used to give pleasure, energy and physical **stimulation**. These effects are usually short-lived; the long-term effects, however, are often damaging. Physically, some drugs can destroy the person's body and mind. People who take illegal drugs on a regular basis may take to crime to provide the cash to support their habit.

There are many different illegal drugs; some of the more commonly used are shown in the table on page 132, with some of their effects and side effects.

Word check

dependency – relying on.
cold turkey – phase that drug addicts go through when they give up drugs; withdrawal symptoms.

Word check

stimulation – arousal or excitement.

Misused drug	Possible effects	Dangers
Cannabis or hash, draw, ganja, marijuana, spliff, weed	• craving for food • feeling anxious • more alert and talkative • lack of energy	• impairs concentration • tiredness, lack of energy • anxiety, paranoia • respiratory disease and lung cancer in long-term users
LSD or acid, trips, tabs	• a 'trip' can last up to 12 hours; once started cannot be stopped • disorientation; objects, colours and sounds can be distorted • sense of movement and time speeds up or slows down	• flashbacks can be frightening from a bad 'trip' • can complicate mental health problems • increasing tolerance to the drug
Heroin or H, Henry, smack, gear, horse, junk	• in small doses, user has sense of warmth and well-being • in large doses, user feels drowsy and relaxed • pain relief	• addiction • increasing tolerance to the drug (users have to take it just to feel normal) • death if impure or taken in excess • HIV/AIDS and hepatitis B when sharing needles • damage to veins at the injection sites
Ecstasy or E, XTC, doves (chemical name is MDMA)	• feeling alert and in tune with surroundings • sound, colour and emotions much more intense • ability to dance for hours (effects last up to six hours)	• risk of overheating and dehydration • possible liver and kidney problems • may lead to brain damage
Cocaine or coke, Charlie, snow	• sense of well-being and confidence • effects last roughly 30 minutes • users often crave more	• damage to veins at the injection sites • can cause chest and heart problems that can be fatal • addiction
Crack (cocaine in a smokeable form) or rock wash, stone	• same effects as cocaine, but more intense and a shorter 'high'	• same effects as cocaine, but as 'high' is more intense, it is more difficult to control
Amphetamines or speed, sulph, whiz, uppers	• excitement – the mind races • feeling confident and full of energy	• tiredness/depression • anxiety • long-term use can lead to mental illness and puts strain on the heart • HIV/AIDS and hepatitis B when sharing needles
Solvents or glue, aerosol, petrol, lighter fluid, hairspray	• similar to feeling drunk – thick-head, dizzy, giggly, dreamy • possibilty of hallucinations • effects do not last long	• vomiting, nausea, black-outs • death from heart problems or suffocation • increased risk of accidents • liver and kidney damage in long-term users

Solvents

Solvents are normally used commercially in paints, inks and cleaning fluids. Some are used in medicine, such as in anaesthetics, to make patients unconscious during operations. Most solvents come in the form of a liquid or a gas. They are often readily available to people who abuse them in the following forms:

- solvent-based glues
- dry-cleaning fluids
- paint solvents
- typing correction fluid
- aerosol sprays
- compressed gases (butane)
- petrol (lighter fluid).

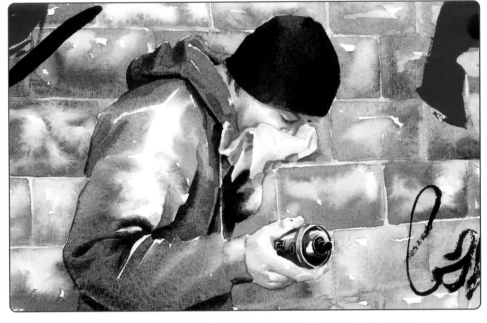

The lining of the nose can be destroyed by this activity

The effect of using these substances can often prove fatal. **Inhaling** solvent gases can severely alter the blood chemistry. This can cause coma and death. The effect of inhaling can cause lung tissue to collapse, which leads to suffocation. Long-term use can lead to liver, kidney and lung failure. Bone marrow and nervous system damage is common and may also be fatal.

Solvent abusers experience **hallucinations** when they may become **disoriented**, which leads to extra danger from everyday hazards such as road traffic. Since these substances have proved to be so dangerous the law regulates their supply. It is an offence under the Intoxicating Substances Supply Act knowingly to supply these substances to any person who might abuse them. It is also an offence to supply them to anyone under the age of 18.

33 Why are solvents dangerous to our health?

People who abuse drugs and solvents are not only a danger to themselves but can be a danger to others as well. There may be a direct risk of violence and increased criminal violence to pay for a drug habit. It is important that we can recognise the signs and symptoms of drug taking. This may allow us to help other people and protect ourselves.

Word check

inhale – breathe in.

Word check

hallucination – seeing things that are not really there.
disoriented – not knowing which direction to take, or what is happening.

Legal substances

Apart from general medications, tobacco and alcohol are the two main legal substances available in this country. Both these substances have the potential to cause major health problems if they are abused.

Tobacco

In recent years tobacco has become less socially acceptable in the UK. Its use has therefore dropped considerably. In the mid 1990s almost 30% of adults were smokers. This led to over 120 000 smoking-related deaths. All these deaths could have been prevented simply by not smoking. Many diseases and medical problems are caused by smoking, including:

- lung cancer
- throat and larynx cancer
- kidney and bladder cancer
- **bronchitis** and **emphysema**
- coronary heart disease
- stroke
- high blood pressure.

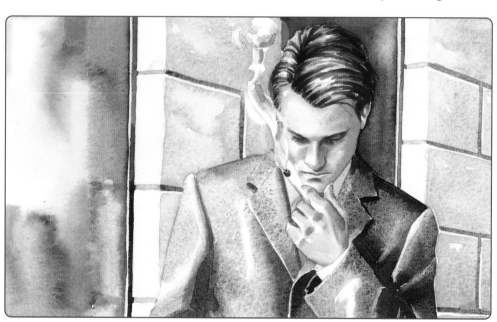

Smoking is legal but less socially acceptable

Word check

nicotine – a stimulant chemical found in cigarettes.

carbon monoxide – poisonous gas.

tar – thick, oily, poisonous substance.

Word check

artery – a blood vessel that carries blood away from the heart.

So what makes smoking so risky? Our bodies suffer the effects of **nicotine**, **carbon monoxide** and **tar**. The dangers are not only confined to the smoker. If we breathe in the smoke from someone else's cigarette we are also at risk. This is known as passive smoking and can increase our risk of getting diseases associated with smoking. When we smoke, the chemicals that are in cigarettes are absorbed into the blood.

Carbon monoxide

In our red blood cells is a substance called haemoglobin which carries oxygen around the body. Carbon monoxide is dangerous because it takes the place of oxygen and takes a long time to be removed. The lack of oxygen can slow body growth and affect heart function. It can also lead to fat being deposited on the artery walls, causing them to harden. This is known as coronary **artery** disease and is the primary heart disease.

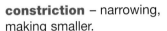

Nicotine

Cigarettes also contain nicotine. This is a fast-acting brain stimulant that has an effect lasting about seven minutes. Nicotine is addictive and leaves the smoker wanting more. This powerful drug causes some immediate effects:

- increase in blood pressure
- increase in heart rate
- **constriction** of small blood vessels
- thickening of blood (leading to increased risk from blood clots)
- change in appetite (usually decreases).

Cigarettes, therefore, can have a harmful effect on the heart, blood and circulation.

> **Word check** ✔
>
> **constriction** – narrowing, making smaller.

Tar

When a cigarette burns it produces a product known as tar. This contains thousands of different chemicals, some of which are carcinogens. Carcinogenic chemicals have the ability to cause cancer.

Tar also damages the small hairs (cilia) that help remove small particles from our lungs. This damage increases our risk of infection and is the reason why smokers are more likely to get chest and throat infections. It also makes conditions like **asthma** and bronchitis worse.

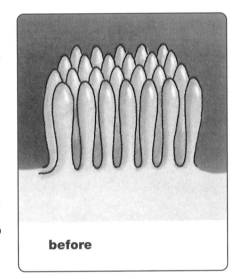

before

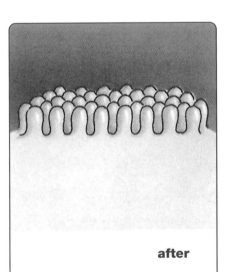

after

Damage to cilia caused by smoking

34 What diseases can you get from smoking?

Smoking and pregnancy

Pregnant women are advised not to smoke as it can harm their unborn child. Smoking can lead to a higher risk of miscarriage. Babies born to mothers who smoke will have a lower weight at birth and be more likely to get chest infections. The risk of sudden infant death syndrome (SIDS) or cot death may also be increased.

> **Word check** ✔
>
> **asthma** – lung disease that makes you short of breath.

35 What does nicotine do to people who smoke?

Smoking places a huge burden on our health care services. This is why the UK government levies such high taxes on tobacco. Smoking is a primary cause of diseases and illnesses that need not happen.

Alcohol

Many people enjoy drinking alcohol. In small amounts, alcohol can give people a lot of pleasure but we must remember that it can still act as a poison.

So, how are we affected by alcohol? Alcohol acts as a **sedative** on the brain. A small amount will reduce the drinker's inhibitions, making them less shy and more relaxed. Most adults can control their intake of alcohol in social situations. However, drinking large amounts of alcohol can affect our self-control because it is also a **depressant**. This can lead to socially unacceptable behaviour, such as fighting or a lack of control of our bodily functions in public, for example vomiting.

People who have drunk a large amount of alcohol often slur their words, lose concentration and stagger around. This is because their muscle control has been affected. A person who is drunk may have blurred vision and may become unconscious. Those who drink large amounts on a regular basis can build up a level of **tolerance**. This means that they show less effects than someone who rarely drinks. Inexperienced drinkers are very much at risk because of their low tolerance. A single session of alcohol abuse can severely damage health and even result in death.

36 What effects does alcohol have on our body?

How the body deals with alcohol

When we drink, the stomach absorbs the alcohol into the blood. When the blood travels through the liver as much alcohol as possible is extracted. This is because the liver changes the alcohol into a substance that it can use for energy. Any that remains is passed out of our bodies in our urine or sweat. Alcohol is a difficult substance for the liver to deal with. The alcohol that the liver cannot burn as energy has to be stored. This means that excessive drinking can cause weight gain – a 'beer gut' can be the result.

> **Word check** ✓
>
> **sedative** – something that makes you sleepy.
> **depressant** – a drug that slows down bodily function.

> **Word check** ✓
>
> **tolerance** – the body needs more of a drug to have the same effect.

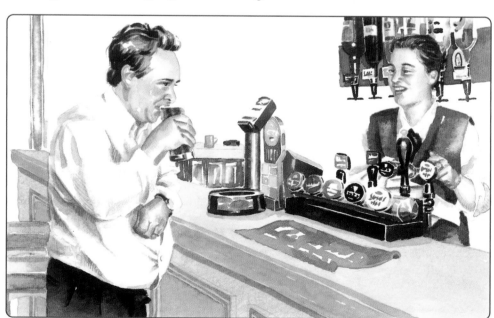

Regularly drinking too much alcohol can affect our health

Is alcohol a risk to health?

Too much alcohol on a regular basis can cause liver damage. This is called **cirrhosis**. The liver also builds up larger than normal amounts of fat which can contribute to liver failure.

There are other health risks from excessive regular drinking, such as:

- high blood pressure
- coronary heart disease
- mouth and throat cancer
- depression (emotional and psychological problems)
- obesity.

A little alcohol, however, can have beneficial properties. Scientists have shown that people who regularly drink small amounts of alcohol, live longer than people who do not drink at all. It must be remembered that alcohol affects different people in different ways. Some people find alcohol addictive. An addiction to alcohol is known as alcoholism.

> **Word check** ✓
>
> **cirrhosis** – a disease that damages the liver, can be caused by alcohol.

Blood alcohol (mg/100ml)	Effects on the average drinker
20	Feeling good; little or no effect on performance
40	Able to let go socially; on top form
60	Judgment impaired; incapable of making important decisions
80	Definite loss of coordination; unsafe driving at any speed
100	Tendency to lose sexual control; knocking over drinks
160	Obviously drunk; possibly aggressive; unmanageable; may have later loss of memory of events
300	Often lose control of bladder and bowels; barely awake; may be in a coma
500	Liable to die without medical attention

Effects of drinking alcohol

In 1997, the World Health Organisation concluded that the reduced risk from coronary heart disease was found at the level of one drink, consumed every second day. In small amounts alcohol helps to reduce blood cholesterol, a substance that can cause heart disease and heart attacks. It also helps us maintain lower fat levels in our blood, which aids our circulation.

Cholesterol, see page 104

37 What are the risks to the body from drinking alcohol?

One unit of alcohol is generally recognised as:

- one small glass (125ml) of wine
- half a pint (285ml) of beer
- one pub measure of spirits.

However, the alcohol content of different drinks does vary. Some strong beers and lagers may contain as much as 2.5 units of alcohol in each half pint. We must remember that measures of spirits poured at home are usually bigger than pub measures. Cans of beer and lager often contain about three-quarters of a pint, rather than half a pint, and so one can contains 1.5 units of alcohol. This can be more if the drink is high strength.

Social drinking can be a pleasurable experience. It is an opportunity to get together with friends, relatives or work colleagues. We need to be careful to stay within the safe limits for drinking alcohol.

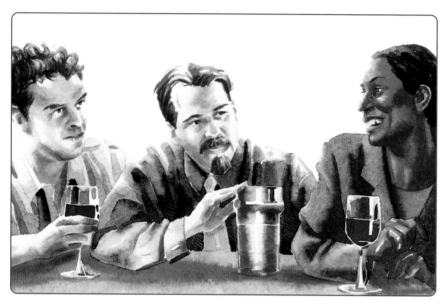

Social drinking can be pleasurable

Finding out about risks to health   ACTIVITY

A1 Make a list of the short- and long-term health risks linked to smoking.

A2 Draw up a plan to show how a person who smokes could be helped to give up.

A3 Find out the safe limits of alcohol for men and women.

A4 Draw up a plan to help a person, who is drinking too much alcohol on a regular basis, to reduce their alcoholic intake.

A5 Using the table on the next page, work out how many Calories are in a one-litre bottle of sweet white wine.

A6 What are the short- and long-term risks to health and well-being of drinking too much alcohol on a regular basis?

A7 Whole group discussion:

- Why you think people take drugs.

- Has society's view of drug-taking changed in the last five years? See if you can find any additional information to support your views.

A8 Carry out some research to find out about TWO organisations that could provide support for alcoholics or drug users who want to kick the habit.

The safety limits for drinking alcohol that have been set by scientists are different for men and women. British recommendations for women are not to exceed two or three units of alcohol per day, and for men are three or four units of alcohol per day. The table below shows the number of Calories in a drink containing one unit of alcohol. Someone on a diet might want to avoid drinking strong ale.

We all need to be aware that alcoholism is increasing. Drinking too much alcohol on a regular basis can be a major health hazard.

It must be remembered that drinking any alcohol can affect the ability to drive. It is our moral responsibility not to drink and drive.

Calorific values of alcoholic drink

Type of drink	Number of Calories in one unit of alcohol
Bitter, can or draught	91
Bitter, keg	88
Mild on draught	71
Brown ale	80
Pale ale	91
Stout	105
Strong ale (special brew)	205
Lager (premium)	85
Sweet cider	110
Dry cider	95
Red wine	85
Rosé wine, medium	89
Sweet white wine	118
Dry white wine	83
Medium white wine	94
Sparkling white wine	95
Port	79
Sherry, dry	58

One unit of alcohol for beers, lager and cider is a half pint (285ml)
One unit of alcohol for wines is a small glass (125ml)
One unit of alcohol for fortified wines is 50ml

Sexually transmitted diseases

As we grow we all develop needs and desires. It is a normal part of our genetic make up to want to be with people. Sexual relationships are just another one of our needs. The need is triggered by the hormone changes in our body. There is also the **fundamental** need for us to keep the human race going. This is our desire to have children of our own. Human beings are believed to be the only animals to have sexual intercourse for pleasure. This is because we have developed higher mental abilities and the power of decision-making.

> **Word check** ✓
>
> **fundamental** – basic.

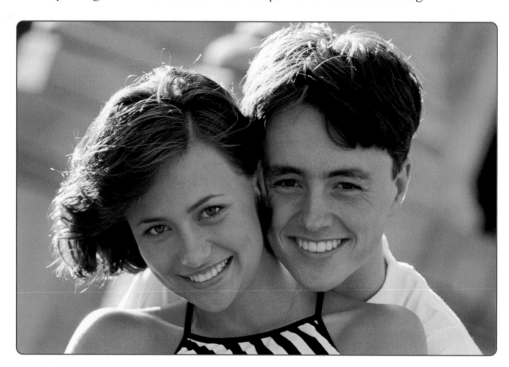

Being in love means being responsible, too

> **Word check** ✓
>
> **abstinence** – avoidance, not taking part in; saying no.

Choosing to have a sexual relationship can involve a certain amount of risk to our health and well-being. The two main areas of risk are unwanted pregnancy and sexually transmitted infections (STIs). Both of these can be reduced by avoiding unprotected sex. This can be through **abstinence**, which means not having sex at all. Alternatively we can use a contraceptive. Barrier methods, such as a condom or femidom, prevent conception and reduce the risk of infection. Barrier methods reduce both risks but are not totally reliable.

The biggest danger from unprotected sex is sexually transmitted infections. Research has shown that the people most at risk from STIs are aged between 15 and 30. This is probably because people are in and out of relationships more between these ages. It does not matter whether you are **heterosexual**, **homosexual** or **bisexual**, the risk is still there. It may only take one single act of unprotected sex to become infected.

> **Word check** ✓
>
> **heterosexual** – someone who forms a sexual relationship with a member of the opposite sex.
>
> **homosexual** – someone who forms a sexual relationship with a member of the same sex.
>
> **bisexual** – someone who has sexual relationships with both male and female partners.

38 What are the risks from having unprotected sex?

There are over 30 different types of STI that affect over 1 million men and women in the UK every year (approximately one in every 65 people). This list shows the ten most common types of STI.

- HIV/AIDS
- syphilis
- gonorrhoea
- non specific urethritis (NSU)
- hepatitis
- chlamydia
- thrush
- genital herpes
- genital warts
- pubic lice

The STI table in the Appendix (page 270) makes it easier for us to see the effects that they can have on our health.

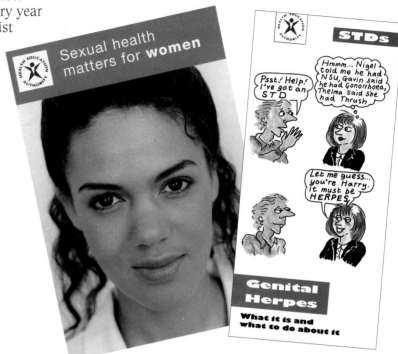

STI	What to watch for	How do you get this STI?	What can happen?
Chlamydia	• Symptoms usually appear 7–21 days after infection. Many women and some men have no symptoms.	• Vaginal or anal sex with someone who has chlamydia.	• YOU CAN GIVE CHLAMYDIA TO YOUR SEXUAL PARTNER(S). • Can lead to a more serious infection.

Appendix 8, see page 270

Three out of the list of ten are life threatening if left untreated.

HIV and AIDS

HIV (human immuno-deficiency virus) is the **virus** that people become infected with. AIDS (acquired immuno-deficiency syndrome) is the problem that the virus causes. As the name suggests, it totally destroys our immunity to other diseases. This means that even the common cold can be fatal to a sufferer in the latter stages of AIDS.

AIDS is one of the worst **pandemics** the world has ever known. HIV, the virus that causes AIDS, was first discovered in 1981 in a remote area of central Africa. It has since swept across the globe, infecting millions in a relatively short period of time. AIDS has killed 21.8 million people that we know of, with 3 million people dying in the year 2001 alone. Currently 40 million people in the world are living with AIDS. While many cases go unreported, the disease is increasing. To illustrate the size of the problem, imagine if one in every three people in the UK were to die. This would be the same number of people that have died of AIDS worldwide by 2003.

Word check

virus – group that are much smaller than bacteria and are likely to be harmful.

Word check

pandemic – disease occurring worldwide.

HIV/AIDS statistics

Number of people affected worldwide by HIV/AIDS	
People newly infected with HIV in 2001	Total 5 million
Adults Of which women Children <15 years	4.2 million 2 million 800 thousand
Number of people living with HIV/AIDS in 2001	Total 40 million
Adults Of which women Children <15 years	37.1 million 18.5 million 3 million
AIDS deaths in 2001	Total 3 million
Adults Of which women Children <15 years	2.4 million 1.1 million 580 thousand
Total number of AIDS deaths since the beginning of the epidemic until 2001	Total 21.8 million
Adults Of which women Children <15 years	17.5 million 9 million 4.3 million
Total number of AIDS orphans since the beginning of the epidemic until the end of 2001	Total 14 million

Source: World Health Organisation

Many people who have the HIV virus, have no visible symptoms of illness. They can live healthy lives for many years after infection. This is because the virus can remain inactive for as much as six to ten years.

39 What is the difference between HIV and AIDS?

How do people get HIV? There are three main ways.

- Unprotected sex (vaginal or anal), this will involve contact with infected body fluids (**semen**, vaginal fluids). By not using condoms or other barriers during sex the risk is greatly increased.

- Infected blood: drug users who share needles; direct contact with infected blood and blood products.

- Pregnancy. During pregnancy and before and after the birth, the virus can be passed on to the baby. The virus can even be passed on by breastfeeding the baby.

At present there is no known cure for HIV/AIDS, but there is hope that a vaccine will be available in the near future.

Hepatitis

There are seven known hepatitis viruses; the main one that is sexually transmitted is Hepatitis B. It is spread in a similar way to HIV, by unprotected sex and blood contact. If left untreated the virus can lead to liver cancer and

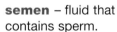

Word check

semen – fluid that contains sperm.

liver failure, both of which can be fatal. A **vaccine** against the virus is available and gives protection for up to five years. Babies born to mothers who are Hepatitis B positive have a 95% chance of contracting the disease. The symptoms of this disease appear within 40 days to six months of being infected. The symptoms include tiredness, abdominal pain, loss of appetite, nausea and vomiting, dark urine, diarrhoea and jaundice.

40 How is hepatitis transmitted?

Syphilis

This is a disease that is transmitted by unprotected sex and can develop in three stages. The first stage leads to sores developing in various areas like the tongue, lips, mouth or genitals. These will heal without treatment, giving a false impression that the problem has gone. However, within weeks or months the second stage will start spreading throughout the body. Painless skin rashes appear and disappear. Fever develops with headaches and hair loss.

If left untreated the third (tertiary) stage develops. Lesions that destroy the skin begin to appear. The heart muscle is affected leading to heart attack. The nervous system is also attacked, possibly leading to dementia.

The disease can be treated in the first two stages with antibiotics but in the later stages it can be impossibe to treat effectively.

Babies born to a mother infected with syphilis have a high chance of being born with the disease. They may also have other associated problems and can be born blind.

Less serious STIs

Other STIs that are more common and less dangerous are thrush and chlamydia. Thrush is a fungal infection caused by an organism called Candida. It appears as a thick white discharge, causing itching, soreness, swelling and pain. Chlamydia can cause more serious problems such as pelvic inflammatory disease (PID). This can lead to inflammation of the **fallopian tubes**. The symptoms can be pain on passing water and irregular bleeding. As it is caused by bacteria it can be transferred on the fingers, and can lead to infections in other areas such as the eyes.

41 List ten STIs.

All sexually contracted infections affect our lives whether it is socially, emotionally or physically. They also have an effect on the lives of others. People do not get these diseases without having sexual contact. What we must remember is that a number of these diseases can prove fatal. They are all preventable and all it takes is safe sexual practice, common sense and education. When it comes to safe practice we should 'spread the word not the disease'.

Sexual behaviour — ACTIVITY

A1 List three risks to health from having unprotected sex.

A2 Why is safe sexual practice important?

A3 Design a leaflet to give advice about safe sex. Make sure that it contains the important points that you think people need to know.

The effects of stress on health

Stress can be caused by worry. We may be unhappy about our friends or home life, our job or personal relationships. The psychological effects of worry can lead to physical problems. Stress can:

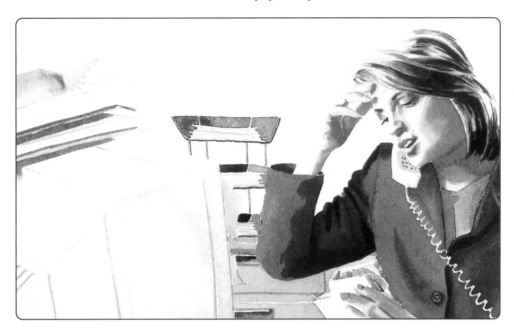

Are you stressed?

- affect sleeping patterns, appetite and emotions

- make us irritable or depressed

- cause panic/anxiety attacks, twitching, chest pains and breathing difficulties, even vomiting, **diarrhoea** and sickness

- lower our resistance to infection because it depresses the immune system

- raise our blood pressure.

Word check

adrenaline – a hormone that stimulates the body to be alert.

Word check

diarrhoea – loose or fluid bowel movement.

Word check

aggravate – make worse.

Word check

depression – feeling very unhappy, or despondent.

When you are under stress, your body produces the hormone **adrenaline**. It mobilises fatty acids that provide us with a source of energy. This is why exercise is important and helps relieve stress.

Many people suffer from skin diseases that are brought on, or **aggravated**, by stress. These can take the form of a rash or small bumps known as hives. Stress can also be a factor that causes, or aggravates, acne. Red, scaly patches known as psoriasis can affect your skin, scalp, elbows, knees and back. These health trends tend to run in families but attacks can be triggered by stress.

Eczema, which gives you itchy, dry skin or sore, weeping blisters commonly gets worse at times of stress. This can happen when you are facing examinations, starting college or a new job or adjusting to different situations.

42 How can stress affect us?

Stress can lead to periods of **depression**. Stress also has a major effect on the heart and circulation. The increase in chemicals like adrenaline can cause your blood pressure to rise. This is why too much stress can lead to heart attacks and strokes as we get older. If we allow stress continuously to affect our lives it can be a killer.

43 Why can stress be a killer?

Personal hygiene

Personal cleanliness promotes our good health and well-being. Regular washing and attention to our personal hygiene helps to control the growth of bacteria, viruses and fungi. Left uncontrolled, some of these **organisms** could cause disease and illness. Our body provides an ideal breeding ground for some of these organisms. This is because we are warm and produce moisture in the form of sweat. Also in our sweat are waste products and dead cells that can provide ideal growing conditions for bacteria. There are few areas of our body where we do not sweat. This means that most areas need cleaning, especially where we have hair and keep constantly clothed.

> **Word check**
>
> **organism** – life form.

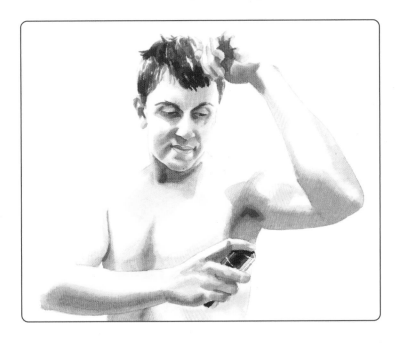

When we are near other people it is important not smell sweaty

Lack of personal hygiene can be a difficult social problem that can lead to exclusion from group activities. If we allow bacteria to build up on our skin we may start to smell. This is socially unacceptable. In some other countries body odour does not carry such social stigma.

Becoming infectious

We can pass on dangerous diseases and infections. It is important to have good toilet hygiene, for example, washing our hands after going to the lavatory. In our gut we all carry bacteria that are capable of causing food poisoning. **Listeria** and **E. coli** are commonly found in the human gut where they are part of our digestive process. By not washing our hands we can unknowingly spread harmful bacteria.

> **Word check**
>
> **Listeria** – type of bacterium.

Anyone who is already ill or unwell has a much greater risk from illnesses such as food poisoning. In certain situations where the person is already seriously ill this can prove fatal.

> **Word check**
>
> **E. coli** – type of bacterium.

Mass outbreaks of food poisoning are fortunately rare in the UK. However, when they do occur they can usually be traced back to poor hygiene.

44 **Why is it important to wash your hands after going to the lavatory?**

Dental hygiene

Why is it important to brush our teeth regularly?

Bacteria are found in the mouth. This is quite normal. Saliva helps to stop bacteria building up when we are chewing. At other times the bacteria produce an acid, which can build up around the teeth and in food particles. When this happens, small areas of tooth enamel can be dissolved. This is how cavities are created and where tooth decay can start. If this carries on it will break into the **pulp cavity** of the tooth. The nerve in the tooth will become irritated and we experience toothache. By brushing our teeth regularly we can give them a higher level of protection.

Maintaining a good level of personal hygiene is very important. Many diseases and infections can be **eradicated** or controlled by good personal hygiene practice.

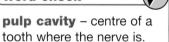

Word check

pulp cavity – centre of a tooth where the nerve is.

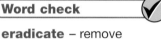

Word check

eradicate – remove completely.

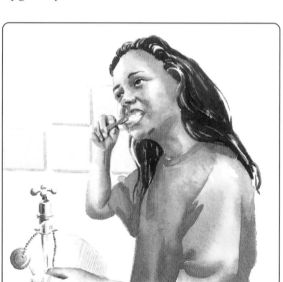

Oral hygiene is very important

Social class and poverty

Social class determines our position in society. Thirty years ago we would have defined people by their class:

- upper class (the monarchy, royalty, titled people, all those with unearned income)

- middle class (professional people such as, doctors, dentists, lawyers, and all other wealthy people)

- lower class (working class, poor).

More recently the government has redefined the class system in this country as is shown in the table. We now have five different classes where title, breeding and wealth have been taken out of the assessment.

Social class	Category	Examples
A or 1	Higher professional and higher managerial	Lawyer, doctor
B or 2	Lower professional and lower managerial	Teacher, farmer, police officer
C or 3	Skilled manual and remainder of non-manual workers	Plumber, clerical worker, mechanic
D or 4	Semi-skilled worker	Lorry driver, postal worker
E or 5	Unskilled worker	Labourer, messenger, cleaner

Source: Registrar-General

Some sociologists do not find the Registrar-General's scale adequate and prefer to use the Hall-Jones scale (see Appendix, page 269) which divides people into seven categories.

It is thought that there is a link between class and health. If a person is in the lower social classes their risk of illness, disease and infection is thought to be increased. This is because poor living conditions and poor diet are more likely to affect a person's health status. Being in the lower social class can even decrease **life expectancy**. It appears to be easier to stay healthy when a person is educated, working and has a reasonable income.

Word check

life expectancy – the average length of time that a person will live.

Appendix 7, see page 269

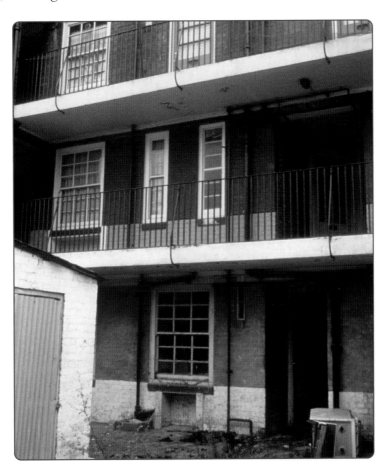

Poor housing can affect our health

Housing and social isolation

Housing or other accommodation can affect health. Cold and damp conditions in the home can aggravate chest problems and conditions such as **arthritis**, **rheumatism**, bronchitis and asthma. In damp conditions **mould** can thrive. As they grow they produce **spores** that can aggravate existing chest problems.

Damp can be especially dangerous for babies and small children. They tend to be the most easily affected by poor living conditions. Overcrowded accommodation may also increase the spread of disease. Where people live closely together infectious diseases often spread more quickly. We all know how a cold can soon spread in a family, even when living in good conditions. In the past when people lived in overcrowded conditions the spread of tuberculosis (TB), cholera and typhoid often reached **epidemic** levels. These diseases were associated with poor living conditions and bad sanitation. Improvements in living conditions have now made these diseases almost unheard of in the UK.

45 Why is good quality housing important?

Our home environment plays a big part in influencing our health and well-being. People who live in high-rise tower blocks can suffer from **social isolation**. The design of such flats means people rarely see their neighbours. They have no sense of belonging to a community. This is a particular problem for young mothers and older adults, who may have to rely on the lifts in the building. If the lifts fail then they can feel trapped.

If a person is immobile or has a small child in a pushchair they can find it a major problem to get down ten fights of stairs and so they may become isolated from friends and family. This type of isolation can often lead to depression, low self-esteem and in severe cases the contemplation of suicide.

The government now realises that the large number of high-rise flats that were built in the 1960s, could have been a mistake. The long-term plan is to make housing more community-centred. High-rise flats are now being demolished to be replaced by accommodation that does not go above four floors.

46 Why do people often feel isolated in high-rise flats?

47 What are the effects of social isolation?

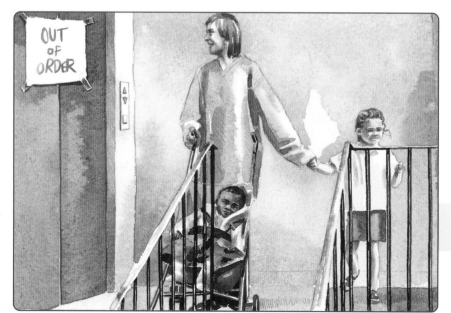

I'll stay in today – I can't face those stairs

Environmental pollution

In the UK we are lucky enough to live in a relatively unpolluted environment. Or do we?

What types of pollution are there? They include:

- air pollution
- water pollution
- waste and litter
- noise.

Air pollution

Clean air is essential to our survival as it supplies us with the oxygen our bodies need to live. Human activities in places such as factories can release dangerous substances into the air, that can cause health problems.

Effects of air pollution include smog, **acid rain**, the **greenhouse effect**, and 'holes' in the **ozone layer**.

Air pollution can be caused by the release of **particulates** into the air from burning fuel. Diesel exhaust, for example, contains particulate matter. The particles are very small, measuring about 2.5 micrometres or about 0.0001 inches.

The exhaust from burning fuels in cars, homes and industry is a major source of pollution in the air.

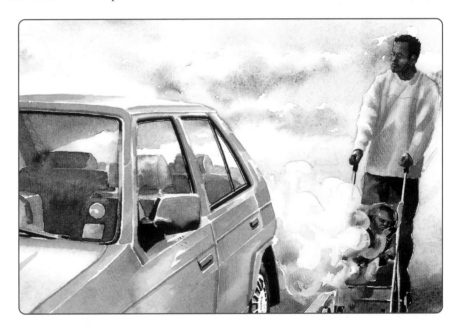

Air quality is affected by the release of **toxic** gases, such as sulphur dioxide, carbon monoxide, nitrogen oxides and chemical vapours. Air pollutants can take part in further chemical reactions once they are in the atmosphere, for example, forming smog and acid rain.

48 What are the main types of pollution?

Health effects of air pollution

Air pollution can affect our health in many ways, with both short- and long-term effects. People are affected by air pollution in different ways. Some people are much more sensitive to pollutants than are others. Young children and older adults often suffer more from the effects of air pollution. People with health problems such as asthma or lung disease may also suffer more when the air is polluted. This is because the pollutants in the air cause a reaction in their lungs, making the smaller airways constrict, so breathing then becomes more difficult.

> **Word check**
>
> **acid rain** – rain that is acidic due to mixing with sulphur dioxide gas pollution.
> **greenhouse effect** – heating effect on the atmosphere.
> **ozone layer** – layer of gas that protects the planet from the sun's harmful rays.
> **particulate** – microscopic particle.

Using our cars causes pollution

> **Word check**
>
> **toxic** – poisonous.

Word check

respiratory – related to the process of breathing.

Word check

chronic – constant or continuing for a long time.

Short-term health effects

Short-term effects can include irritation to the eyes, nose and throat, and upper **respiratory** infections such as bronchitis and pneumonia. Other symptoms can include headaches, nausea, and allergic reactions. Short-term air pollution can aggravate medical conditions like asthma and emphysema. In London in 1952, 4000 people died in a few days due to the high concentrations of pollution, which formed smog. Smog is a dangerous combination of smoke and fog. Fortunately it is now rarely seen in the UK.

Long-term health effects

These can include **chronic** respiratory disease, lung cancer, heart disease, and even damage to the brain, nerves, liver or kidneys. Continual exposure to air pollution affects the lungs of growing children and may complicate medical conditions in older adults.

49 What is smog?

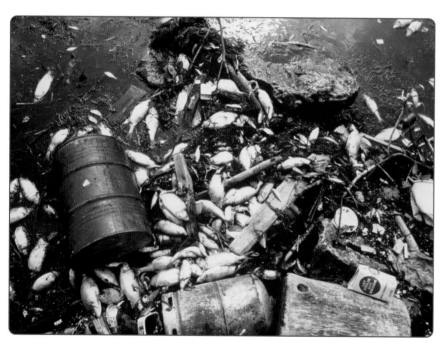

The fish are dead; the water is polluted

Water pollution

Clean water is essential for healthy living. Fresh, clean drinking water is a basic need for all people. The main source of freshwater pollution is from discharge of untreated waste, dumping of industrial **effluent**, and run-off from fertilisers from agricultural fields. In urban areas water can be contaminated from leaking water pipe joints and broken sewage pipes.

Water-borne infectious diseases include hepatitis, cholera, dysentery and typhoid, but these are unlikely to occur in the UK. Exposure to polluted water can cause diarrhoea, skin irritation, respiratory problems and other diseases. The symptoms depend on the pollutant that is in the water.

Water-borne health hazards are mainly due to incorrect management of water resources. Proper management of water resources will ultimately lead to a cleaner and healthier environment. In order to prevent the spread of water-borne infectious disease, water supplies should be properly checked and necessary steps taken to disinfect them. In the UK we often add chemicals like chlorine and fluorine to our water. These help disinfect our water supplies. If there is any doubt about the cleanliness of our water supply we should boil water before we use it.

50 Why is clean water important?

Word check

effluent – sewage and waste water.

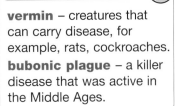

Waste and litter

Most of us have been guilty at some time of dropping litter and some of us probably still do. Stop for a moment and imagine what the country would look like if we all did it. There would be endless piles of rubbish. Just imagine how many bags of rubbish your family produces in one week. Now multiply that by 30 million. This will give you an idea of the amount of household rubbish that is produced in the UK. Side by side the bags would cover the city of Birmingham and there would still be plenty left over. The amount of commercial rubbish produced is even greater.

This may indicate how important it is to our health to dispose of rubbish correctly. Discarded rubbish leads to the spread of diseases. It attracts flies and rats and other dangerous **vermin**. Rats have been especially harmful in the past. This is because they were the cause of many outbreaks of **bubonic plague**. Athough this killer disease has not occurred for over 200 years, rats still carry diseases that are harmful to humans.

We are all responsible for stopping pollution. Sensible actions on our part help maintain our good health. Being tidy and recycling improve our well-being by protecting our environment.

51 Why can litter and rubbish be dangerous to our health?

> **Word check** ✓
>
> **vermin** – creatures that can carry disease, for example, rats, cockroaches.
> **bubonic plague** – a killer disease that was active in the Middle Ages.

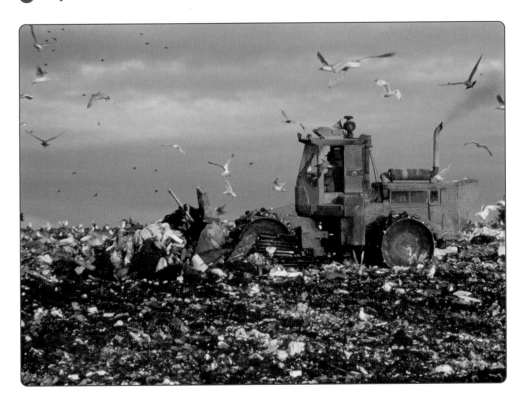

Rubbish pollutes our environment

Noise pollution

Noise can be damaging to our health, particularly if we regularly experience noise that is above an acceptable level. It is not just our ears that are affected by noise pollution, but our whole nervous system, including the brain.

Noise pollution occurs in a variety of ways. It can be self-inflicted through wearing headphones to listen to music at high volume, or by having the television or radio on so loud that eventually our ears are damaged.

Noise can affect us if we live near a busy main road where there is constant traffic, or near an airport where aircraft are departing and arriving throughout the day and night. The noise from vehicles and aircraft can make us feel irritable. We may feel we have no peace and quiet in which to think and make rational decisions. Being irritable can upset the people around us, because we become short-tempered. This could result in losing friends and becoming more isolated. This would affect our social and emotional well-being.

In today's society, noise is a form of pollution that is steadily increasing.

Risks to health and well-being · ACTIVITY

A1 You are working in a residential home for older adults. List FIVE ways that your own personal hygiene can be maintained.

A2 Describe how infection can be spread when:

- preparing food

- caring for people who have infections.

A3 Explain how social class can affect health and well-being.

A4 Pat lives in a rural area. There are few buses, and travel to the town is expensive.

- Describe why Pat may feel socially isolated.

- What are the likely effects of social isolation on Pat?

A5 Group discussion:

- Who do you think is responsible for pollution in this country?

- How could pollution be reduced?

A6 Explain the effects of pollution on individuals.

Gillian **CASE STUDY**

Gillian is 13. She lives with her parents and three brothers in a three bedroom flat. The flat is on the ninth floor of a large block. Gillian shares her room with her younger brother who is seven and has asthma. In winter the walls of the room occasionally grow mould and her brother's asthma gets worse. Gillian often fights with her brother.

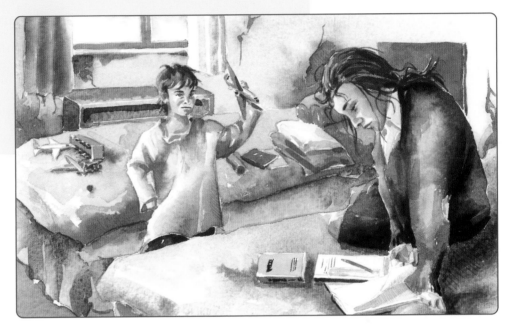

Gillian and her brother have to share a bedroom

Supporting Gillian **ACTIVITY**

A1 What environmental reasons might cause Gillian to fight with her brother?

A2 Gillian's brother's asthma is worse in winter. Give environmental reasons for this.

A3 Why does mould grow on the walls of the flat?

A4 Draw up a plan for Gillian and her brother to help them improve their health.

A5 Carry out research to find some leaflets that would provide support for Gillian and her family. Explain how the leaflets you have chosen would help the family.

Indicators of physical health

Getting started

How can an individual's physical health be measured?

Some indicators of physical health can be measured. They are used to see how physically healthy people are. There are a variety of methods of assessing physical health. Many of them you can perform yourself. 'High tech' equipment is not always necessary and often you can get your results using simple scientific methods.

This could be something as basic as taking someone's temperature or comparing their weight against their height.

In this section you will:

- find out how to measure blood pressure
- find out how to measure peak flow
- learn about body mass index
- learn how to measure resting pulse and recovery after exercise
- understand that a person's age, sex and lifestyle affect the results that are obtained when measuring physical health.

Measuring blood pressure is one form of assessment

Measuring our health

We have looked at a variety of factors that influence our health. Health can be measured, but how?

When we visit the GP or hospital a whole range of tests are available. It is not only professionals that can measure health. We can monitor our own health. Here are some measurements that can be taken:

- temperature
- BMI (body mass index)
- height/weight
- peak flow
- recovery rate (after exercise).

When measuring health we will mostly be using conventional **SI units**. When health workers carry out these tasks they refer to them as clinical tests. Health professionals take **physical** and **physiological measurements**. The word physical is applied to basic measurements like weight and temperature.

Physiological measurements show how body **functions** are working. Examples of this are blood pressure and peak flow, both of which we will look at later on (pages 161 and 163). These are more complex and are usually a collection of values. Blood pressure is a good example because it is made up of more than one measurement. It is the measurable force on the vessels that is created when the heart pumps blood around the body. This will vary in different people due to age, weight or illness.

Another method of measuring health is to use charts. These are graphs or tables that provide information. Over the years health care professions have produced various **charts**. Their purpose is to show the **range** of normal readings. These include body mass index and height/weight charts. They measure what is commonly considered to be normal across the population. One of the best examples of this is a height/weight ratio chart. This compares a person's height against their weight. The chart can be used by health care professionals, and by ourselves, to check if we are at the right weight for our height.

Height and weight

The relationship between height and weight can be a good indicator of the state of an adult's health. As a rule our weight should be proportional to our height, but what does this mean? By looking at the whole population scientists have worked out the weight you should be for your height. A person will be considered to be **obese** when their weight is 20% or more above the normal average weight for people of the same height. To make this as accurate as possible scientists based this on individuals with similar personal and cultural characteristics. From this they have produced a general chart that gives a range of comparisons of height against weight.

Word check

SI units – internationally agreed metric units of measurement.
physical measurement – height and weight or other measurement.
physiological measurement – blood pressure, peak flow or measurement of other body function.
function – what something does.

Word check

chart – document containing values and measurements.
range – extent from highest to lowest.

Word check

obese – very overweight.

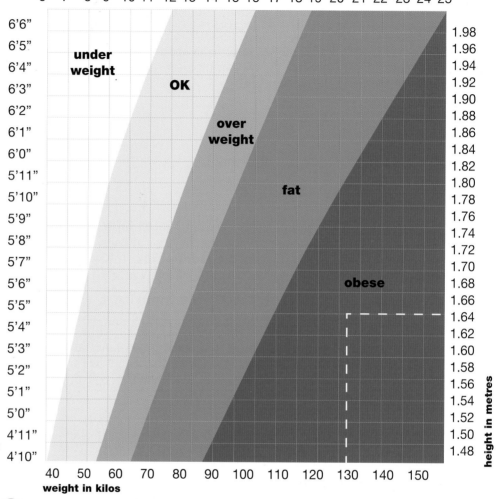

weight in stones

6 7 8 9 10 11 12 13 14 15 16 17 18 19 20 21 22 23 24 25

under weight

OK

over weight

fat

obese

height in feet and inches

6'6" 6'5" 6'4" 6'3" 6'2" 6'1" 6'0" 5'11" 5'10" 5'9" 5'8" 5'7" 5'6" 5'5" 5'4" 5'3" 5'2" 5'1" 5'0" 4'11" 4'10"

height in metres

1.98 1.96 1.94 1.92 1.90 1.88 1.86 1.84 1.82 1.80 1.78 1.76 1.74 1.72 1.70 1.68 1.66 1.64 1.62 1.60 1.58 1.56 1.54 1.52 1.50 1.48

40 50 60 70 80 90 100 110 120 130 140 150
weight in kilos

Word check

category – class or group.

The chart shows **categories** that range from underweight to obese. By reading the two measurements (height and weight) for the person, from the chart, and looking at the point where the two meet, it is possible see exactly in which category they fall. For example, someone who is 1.64m tall and weighs 130kg comes in the obese category, as shown on the chart.

Monitoring health   ACTIVITY

A1 Weigh and measure four of your friends.

- Plot the measurements on a graph that will be provided by your teacher.

- What categories do they fall into?

A2 How can knowing the height and weight measurements help you to work out a health plan for a person?

A3 Look at the example on the chart, for someone weighing 130kg who is 1.64m tall:

- draw up a menu for their breakfast

- show how the menu could help the person reduce their weight.

We have to remember that this method gives us a general picture of our health and status and does not provide a truly accurate or specific picture of our health.

Let us think about a weightlifter, weighing 100kg and 1.80m tall. Our chart would make him fat. But, he needs his weight for the sport he pursues. So there are **exceptions**; this means that we cannot use a single method in **isolation** as it can be inaccurate.

52 What do you understand the word obese to mean?

Body Mass Index (BMI)

Another measurement we could use is **Body Mass Index (BMI)**.

Looking at the height/weight chart we found that our weightlifter seems to be fat. Let us see how he measures up using the BMI test. A BMI is a straightforward calculation that gives an index number. Again, scientists have worked out statistically what the healthy range is. The calculation looks like this.

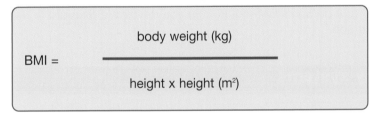

$$BMI = \frac{body\ weight\ (kg)}{height \times height\ (m^2)}$$

In the weightlifter's case he still does not fit into the scientists' category of 'normal', even though we see him as a picture of health.

Working out the weightlifter's BMI

As a weightlifter, the balance of his body tissues is different to that of the average man in the street. He has very little body fat and much more muscle than normal. With his weight at 100kg and his height being 1.80m, the calculation will look like this.

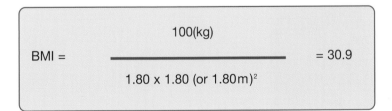

$$BMI = \frac{100(kg)}{1.80 \times 1.80\ (or\ 1.80m)^2} = 30.9$$

30.9 is the body mass index number.

His index number of 30.9 is above the normal range of 20–24 for men (19–24 for women). Having a number over 30 just puts him in the obese range, which we know is incorrect. His body is made up of more muscle than fat which has confused the calculation. This is because most people do not have such a large amount of muscle.

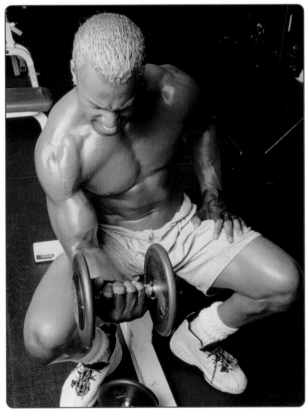

He needs all his strength

Word check

exception – something not like the norm.
isolation – on its own.

Word check

Body Mass Index (BMI) – a scientific calculation that gives an index number that relates to a person's size.

For most people this system works well. This is because the extra weight that we carry is usually fat. Our 'super-fit' weightlifter is an exception.

Calculating BMI

ACTIVITY

 Try calculating your own BMI and compare the results that you get with the table below:

weight group	BMI (kg/m²)	obesity class
underweight	<18.5	
normal	18.5–24.9	
overweight	25.0–29.9	
obesity	30.0–34.9 35.0–39.9	I II
extreme obesity	40.0+	III

A2 Now try calculating the BMI for another person in your group.

A3 Explain how knowing a person's BMI could help you develop a plan of exercise for that person.

Word check ✔

pulse – the wave passing along the arteries each time the heart beats.

Measuring body systems

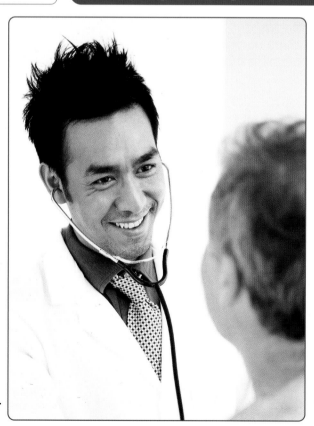

Measuring our body systems is an indicator of how healthy we are

Pulse and breathing rates can provide important information. Looking at these can give us a good overview of a person's health and fitness. So what is our pulse and how do we use it to measure health?

Pulse

We can feel a pulse at many different points on the body. We have probably all seen nurses and doctors taking a pulse. What they are actually doing is pressing a blood vessel called an artery, against something solid like a muscle or bone. The artery in the neck and the one in the wrist are commonly used places. The force of the heart pumping blood around the arteries causes the pulsing sensation that can be felt. We measure this in 'beats per minute' and the only equipment needed is a watch with a second hand.

Health practitioners are usually very busy people. To save time they do not measure the pulse rate for one minute. This is because the heart has a very regular beat so they measure it for 15 seconds, then multiply the number by four. For example,

Pulse rate is 18 beats in 15 seconds.
We need to multiply both by four.

18 beats x 4 = 72 beats;
15 seconds x 4 = 60 seconds (one minute)

The result is 72 beats per minute.

This usually proves to be an accurate way of measuring pulse rate.

Taking a pulse rate measurement   ACTIVITY

A1 Measure a friend's pulse rate for 15 seconds at the point of the wrist. Calculate what the pulse rate will be for one minute.

A2 Now measure their pulse rate over one minute and compare the two results. Are they different?

A3 If the difference is within five beats you have a reasonably accurate reading.

A4 How would you use a pulse rate measurement to help plan an exercise programme for a person?

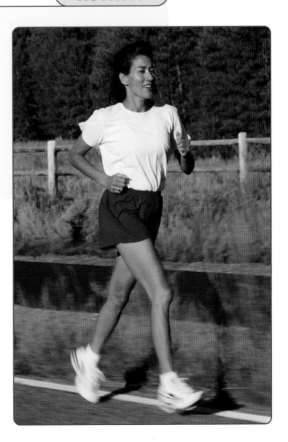

We now have the correct result and we saved 45 seconds. This may not sound much but if you have to check a whole ward of patients the saving soon mounts up. The average adult pulse rate while resting is between 70 and 80 beats per minute. If an adult is very fit it can be as low as 60 beats per minute. A newborn baby's pulse rate can be anything from 120 to as high as 180 beats per minute.

Exercise can reduce our resting pulse rate

When we exercise our pulse rate increases, then returns to normal when we rest. Other events will also cause our pulse rate to increase. For example, if we are scared the brain orders an increase in a chemical called adrenaline. This increases your heart rate and delivers more blood to your body to allow you to act more quickly or run from danger. When the danger is over the brain orders nor adrenaline to be released, to slow your heart down again.

Pulse rate can also be affected by heart disease and lung function. An increase in the rate can be caused by the body not getting enough oxygen. The heart therefore has to pump the oxygen-containing blood around the body much faster.

Recovery rate exercise   ACTIVITY

Health and safety
Tell your teacher if you are usually excused PE because these exercises are unsuitable. If you are asthmatic you should ensure you have your inhaler in case you need it.

A1 Ask someone in the group to record your pulse rate and the number of breaths, for one minute while you are resting.

A2 Exercise for one minute, for example, walk up and down stairs quickly.

A3 Ask your partner to check your pulse rate and number of breaths again immediately after finishing the exercise. Record the results.

A4 Now check your pulse rate every minute until it returns to the resting rate.

A5 Record your results on a table like this:

Name:			
	Pulse rate (beats/min)	Breathing rate (breaths/min)	Recovery rate
Before exercise	84	15	
Exercise finished	120	30	Time starts here
One minute	110	25	
Two minutes	95	20	
Five minutes	84	15	Time stops here 5 mins

The time taken for your pulse to return to normal is known as the recovery rate. It varies for different people and is related to their fitness level – the fitter you are the shorter the recovery time. Recovery time can be improved by regular exercise.

Breathing

All the cells in our body need oxygen to function. This oxygen is collected when we breathe in. When we are resting we breathe in and out at a rate of approximately 20 times in every minute. This is our average breathing rate. As our activity increases so does our breathing rate. This is because activity in the body uses up extra oxygen so we breathe faster.

Illness and disease can affect the rate at which we breathe. Asthma causes a reduction in air flow to the little air sacs (alveoli) in the lungs. This reduces the amount of air getting in and so reduces the amount of oxygen being absorbed. The result is an increase in the rate of breathing. An asthmatic's wheeze is caused by the narrowed airways.

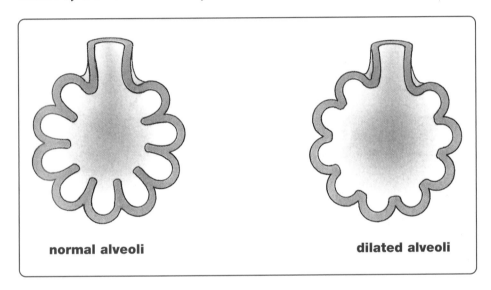

normal alveoli　　　　　**dilated alveoli**

The air sacs can also become too big because of disease known as emphysema. Enlarged air sacs are not an advantage because the surface area that absorbs the oxygen decreases. This causes continuous gasping for air and often the only solution is to use an oxygen mask.

53 What is asthma?

Measuring lung function

Watching someone breathe only gives us basic information. To be more accurate we need to quantify, or give a value to, our measurements. We can do this by using a **peak flow** meter.

This simple machine measures the maximum rate at which you can blow out (expel) air from your lungs in one second. To do this you just breathe out hard. The scale on the side will give your reading in millilitres per second. This can be compared to a table of expected scores. People with chronic lung disease or asthma will normally score below 350 whereas a reasonably fit person will score in the region of 500–600. Very fit athletes can almost blow the needle off of the scale!

> **Word check** ✓
>
> **peak flow** – the maximum rate at which you can expel (blow) air from your lungs.

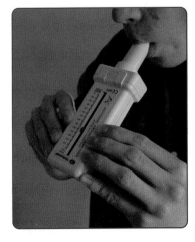

Measuring peak flow

Temperature

Any activity makes you hot but the body is very good at temperature regulation. Within the body a great many complex chemical reactions happen all the time. To make sure that these happen efficiently the human body works to keep the temperature constant at 37 degrees centigrade.

Measuring temperature can often tell us if someone is suffering from an infection, such as the flu (influenza). The virus that causes flu causes a rise in body temperature. This high body temperature is known as **hyperthermia**. This can be dangerous and sometimes fatal. If the temperature inside the body rises too much then organs such as the liver and the brain begin to fail. This can happen if we spend too much time outside in hot weather, or in a hot car, or if we sleep covered by too many blankets. This is why people should not leave babies or young children (or pets) shut in a car on a hot day for any length of time.

Alternatively, if our body temperature falls very low we will suffer from **hypothermia**. With this condition, too, various organs begin to fail and will not function properly. This can affect older people in winter, when they do not have sufficient heating in their homes.

Measuring temperature

Temperature is taken using a clinical thermometer. A clinical thermometer is different from most other thermometers. It is very accurate and can be sterilised to stop the transfer of infection. Some modern thermometers are also disposable. A small disposable thermometer is easier to put under the tongue than other types.

Why do we place the thermometer under the tongue? This is because there are many blood vessels near the skin surface that we can measure. The saliva in our mouth acts as a good conductor of the heat. Keeping the mouth shut keeps in the heat that we are measuring.

Word check ✓

hyperthermia – extremely high body temperature or fever (heat stroke).

hypothermia – condition that develops when the body temperature falls.

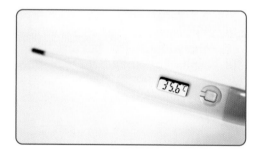

Thermometers tell us what our temperature is

You can also measure temperature rectally using a rectal thermometer. This involves putting the bulb of a specially designed thermometer into the patient's bottom to take the temperature (this should not be attempted by an untrained person). This method is often used in situations where the patient might bite the thermometer, for example, babies. The rectal thermometer is slightly different. It is blue at one end to make it clear which is the correct end to insert.

54 How can you stop infections being transferred when using a non-disposable thermometer?

Blood pressure

Blood pressure (BP) is the measurable force on the vessels that is created when the heart pumps blood around your body. Two measurements are taken when you measure blood pressure. They are known as the systolic pressure and the diastolic pressure. The force of the blood pumping out of the heart creates the systolic pressure. The diastolic pressure is a measurement of the continuous pressure put upon the arteries as the heart relaxes.

Measuring blood pressure

To measure these pressures we use a piece of equipment called a sphygmomanometer, 'sphyg' for short.

A sphygmomanometer consists of an inflatable, soft rubber cuff with an air bladder that is connected to a tube and a bulb. A gauge is used to indicate the air pressure being applied. The gauge is either a column of mercury or, in new equipment, a digital display.

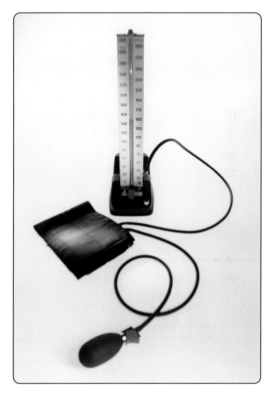

- The cuff of the sphygmomanometer is inflated around the upper arm until it is tight enough to stop the flow of blood through the main artery in the arm.

- The operator uses a stethoscope at the bend of the elbow to check that there is no pulse beating.

- The cuff is then gradually deflated (air let out) until the blood can be heard making its way along the artery (beating).

- A reading is taken and recorded. This is the systolic pressure.

- The cuff is then deflated further (more air let out) until the beat disappears and the blood is flowing steadily through the now open artery.

- A second reading is taken. This gives the diastolic pressure. Blood pressure is recorded as millimetres of mercury (mmHG).

A sphygmomanometer is used to take blood pressure

Blood pressure should only be measured by a trained person, if taken incorrectly, it can be painful and sometimes dangerous.

The average blood pressure of a young, fit person is expected to be about:

$$\frac{120}{80}$$ (120 = systolic, 80 = diastolic)

Doctors will usually judge high blood pressure by taking into account other factors that include height, weight and age.

Stress can be a cause of raised blood pressure. In general it is said that if your systolic pressure is higher than 160 and/or your diastolic is over 100, then you are clinically at risk from high blood pressure. Persistent high blood pressure can lead to problems such as stroke. This is when a small blood vessel in the brain bursts. This causes damage to that area of the brain. If this happens patients can loose the ability to speak and move. A stroke can sometimes cause death.

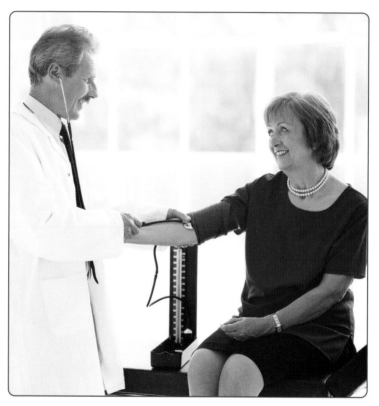

Taking a patient's blood pressure

55 What does a sphygmomanometer measure?

Age, gender and lifestyle

What effects do our age, gender and lifestyle have on our physical health and readings?

Age

As we grow older our body begins to change and so can all the physical values that we have talked about.

- Blood pressure rises with age. At 18 your BP may be 110/65, by the time you are 45 it could be 145/85.

- As we grow older, if we do not maintain our fitness our pulse will rise. At age 18 it may be 60bpm at rest but by age 45 it could be 80bpm.

- Our peak flow may not be so good as we get older. Due to various medical problems it can become lower.

Gender

Gender is often used to refer to the roles of males and females; the ways in which men and women are seen in our society. Gender is the image or picture that we have about the ways in which men and women should behave. Our gender can affect our health and well-being.

- Women store fat in different places to men. This gives us our different shapes.
- Men can be more prone to heart disease and stroke.

Lifestyle

This has the biggest influence of all. Always remember 'you are what you eat', so eat healthily to be healthy. Healthy people with a sensible lifestyle usually:

- maintain the correct weight
- have normal blood pressure
- are fit
- are less prone to disease and infection.

If you are unfit and have a poor lifestyle you may:

- be overweight
- be unfit
- have high blood pressure
- be more prone to infection.

56 How does age affect our blood pressure?

Health assessment ACTIVITY

A1 Choose a person for whom you could make a health plan.

Ask them if you can measure their health. With their agreement obtain the following measurements.

- height
- weight
- pulse rate
- body mass index

- breathing rate
- dietary habits (what they eat and drink)
- how often they exercise
- type of exercise they take.

A2 What do these measurements tell you about the person's health status?

A3 List THREE aspects of their health that they need to improve.

A4 If they need to change anything they are currently doing, how will you convince them to change their habits?

Health promotion and improvement methods

Getting started

How can individuals be motivated and supported to improve their health?

In this section you will learn about the need for realistic assessment, advice and targets in health planning. You will also see how people's behaviour affects their level of target achievement.

In this section you will:

- understand the need for health promotion and information
- understand the benefits of accurate advice and support
- look at methods of assessment and motivation
- understand why planning is important
- show how we can set achievable targets.

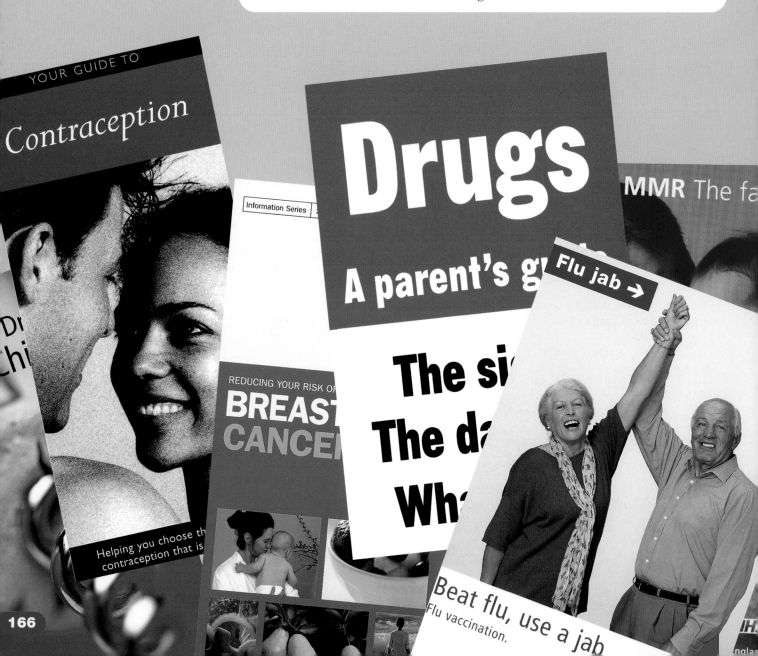

Health promotion and information

Recognising the importance of having good health has lead to active health promotion. It is a good way of providing accurate and helpful information to large numbers of people. Health promotion can make a real difference to the health and well-being of the general public.

We have probably all seen and heard information from health promotion **campaigns** on TV, radio and in newspapers, magazines and pamphlets. These campaigns cover many topics from alcohol and smoking to exercise and obesity. Posters and leaflets advertising ways to achieve good health are all around us – in health centres, leisure centres, schools, colleges and supermarkets.

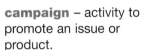

Word check ✓

campaign – activity to promote an issue or product.

This advertising is targeted at groups of individuals of various ages, for example:

- smokers
- drinkers
- young people

- pregnant mothers
- the homeless
- older people.

You will recognise the campaigns aimed at your age group. All campaigns are designed to be eye-catching. It often takes a great deal of money, expertise and effort to make them work.

Health promotion materials   **ACTIVITY**

A1 Look at a selection of FOUR health promotion materials. These can be leaflets, advertisements or any other form of information. Briefly explain the aim of each.

A2 List the audience that each campaign is targeting.

A3 Explain why you think the best ones are effective.

- What catches your eye?

- Are they easy to read?

- Is there a balance between the number of illustrations and the number of words used?

A4 Select one piece of health promotion material. In no more than 50 words explain how it would provide support for a person who is trying to improve their health.

There are many methods that can be used to carry a health promotion message. These include:

- information packs
- posters
- TV, cinema and radio
- booklets and leaflets

- newspapers and magazines
- talks and lectures
- games and role play.

Health assessment and advice

When it comes to assessing a person, everyone's needs are different. Many things will affect a person's ability to take part in health improvement plans. Several factors have to be taken into account.

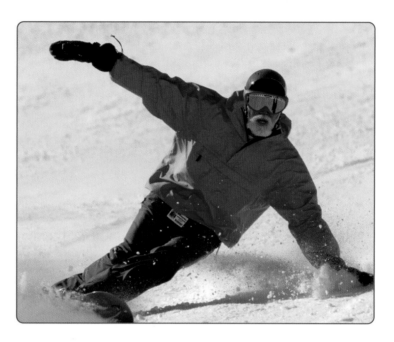

Unless already fit, this activity could be fatal for an older adult

Word check

agility – being able, quick, nimble and active.

- Age, diet and activity have to be suitable – asking someone who is 70 to start cross-country running is neither safe nor suitable.

- Gender – many women do not have the physical strength that men have, but could easily have more **agility**.

- Physical condition – if we have not exercised for a long time we have to start off safely. Gentle exercise to start with can be built up as we get fitter.

- Health condition – we must be careful not to ask people to take part in health plans that might make them worse. If someone is recovering from illness they should seek their doctor's advice before starting on a health improvement plan.

- Social position – many people may not have the time or money to go to a gym. The exercise part of a health plan need only take up a maximum of 30 minutes a day. You do not need special equipment to get fit. A flight of stairs may be enough. People often have to put their family commitments first. They should not be put under pressure to make unacceptable arrangements.

- Motivation – we must want to follow a health plan.

Assessment needs to look at the whole person; this is known as an holistic approach. It has to take account of the person's physical, intellectual, emotional, and social situation (PIES). If we can understand their lifestyle, our assessment is more likely to be successful.

PIES, see pages 9 and 94

Advice

The advice that we give must always be based on our assessment. If we do not do this, our advice could be wrong or prove dangerous. Remember we may not know all the answers. Always be prepared to ask for advice yourself. It is not a failing to ask. Health care professionals do this all the time.

When we advise people we must make sure that:

- they understand the plan
- it is written down (as a plan or description)
- it is suitable (for their age, gender and condition)
- it is accurate
- it is not dangerous and is within their ability.

Once we know what advice to give we can then motivate and support.

57 Why must assessment and advice be accurate?

58 What factors affect the assessment and advice that is given to people?

Motivation and support

Motivation is essential for any plan to improve our condition. The less motivated we are the more we have to rely on willpower; this may work for a little while but it does not always last. It is unlikely to result in long-term successful results. To succeed we must be well motivated. This applies to anyone we are trying to help and especially to ourselves. We must really want to achieve the targets set.

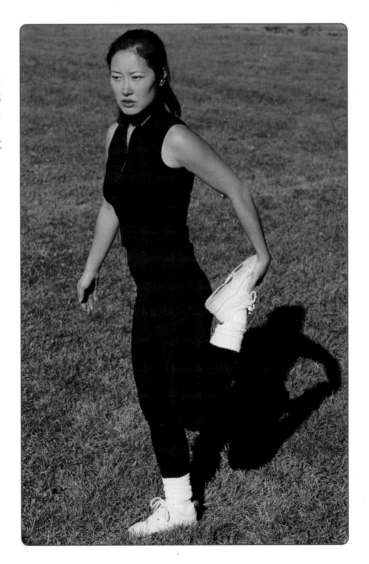

We must want to improve our health

So what is motivation?

Basically it is the reason why we want to succeed. We need to have a really good reason; it needs to be positive and genuine. If we are only doing something because we have been told to do it we are unlikely to succeed. Negative reasons for improving health could include:

- my doctor told me to stop smoking but I enjoy it
- my girlfriend said she would leave me if I did not lose weight.

Good motivation is taking action because we want to. We have a positive reason and it is something we really, really want to do.

- I want to look good for my own sake.
- Being fit will be great.
- My health will improve and I will be able to do so much more with my family.

Keeping a positive attitude is essential to success. If we are motivating and supporting someone else then we have to keep reminding them:

- how well they are doing
- how good they will feel and look when they reach their target
- how much more active they will be

and in the case of giving up smoking:

- how much money they will save.

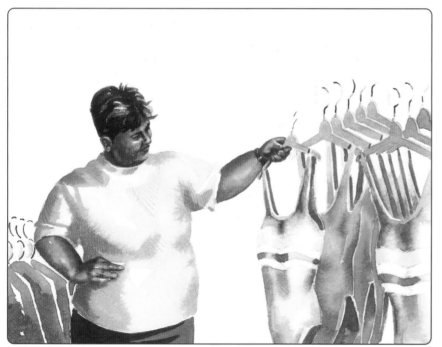

Although some people like to exercise alone, others prefer to be in groups. For these, group activity may be the incentive they need to succeed. Community-based fitness groups often provide the positive support and company that is needed. A little competition from others in the same position can also sometimes help.

Whatever we are trying to do, motivation and support are essential. Being positive can make a major difference to our own goals and the goals of others.

If I swim three times each week I will soon start to look slimmer

59 Describe FIVE different ways of motivating a person to succeed with a health plan.

Planning

Providing people with a good plan to improve their health is very important. When planning, we should remember that the plan should be:

- drawn up with the person so that they feel in control

- accessible – they should be able to do the activities

- achievable – the goals should match the goals of the person and should include short- and long-term targets

- accurate – if you plan something it must be correct

- the goals must be clear – what is the aim?

If we fail in any of these areas then the plan may not work. The biggest motivation for a person is to see results. Even the smallest change for the better can be motivating. This means we should aim for small goals to start with, and bigger ones to follow.

Look at this example of an exercise plan.

Step one	Step two	Step three	Step four
This can last for 2–4 weeks	This can last for 1–2 months	This can last for 1–2 months	This can last for 1–2 months
Stop relying totally on labour-saving devices.	Take a 15-minute walk/swim every day. Do not do any more.	Increase your daily exercise to 20–30 minutes.	Increase your daily exercise to 30 minutes.
Don't rely on your car so much, don't always use the lift, use the stairs.	If bad weather stops you going outside, put on your new CDs and dance for 15 minutes.	Update your exercise diary. Keep a note of your progress and any failures.	Update your exercise diary. Keep a note of your progress and any failures.
While you're getting used to moving around, check out your neighbourhood for possible walks, or a place to exercise, or a swimming pool.	Make a simple exercise diary.	Do not be tempted to do twice the exercise one day and none the next.	Aim gradually to work up to 30-45 minutes of exercise a day.
Ask around and find a friend to start exercising with you.	Persuade a friend/partner to exercise with you.	When you feel ready for more, proceed to Step four.	
Buy a couple of dance music CDs.	When you feel ready for more, proceed to Step three.		
When you feel ready for more, proceed to Step two.			

Setting targets

Setting targets is important. These must be achievable for the person for whom the plan is intended. Unrealistic targets are the biggest reason why health improvement plans fail. The target that is set can be achieved in step-by-step stages. Targets should not be so difficult that they are dangerous. Often a little at a time is best. If the targets are not working, then review them. They may not have been correct in the first place.

By keeping accurate records during the health plan it is possible to monitor what is happening. If a plan begins to fail there has to be a reason. Investigate the reason and see if the problem can be overcome; if necessary modify the plan. This will help the person to get back on track and to succeed.

60 What three 'A's should be considered when drawing up a plan?

Presenting the plan

When presenting a plan to help improve a person's health it must be in a form that they can use, for example:

• a plan for a child should have more pictures than words

• a plan for an older person may need to be in larger print.

Whoever the plan is for it needs to be in a form that they can actually use. For some people this will mean preparing a plan so that it can be placed on a wall where it can be accessed easily. Other people would prefer to have the plan in a booklet. Whichever method is used, the plan needs to look attractive to the user.

Producing a plan   ACTIVITY

A1 Your best friend wants to lose 10 pounds (4.5kg) in weight. You know that she is not a healthy eater and she takes very little exercise. Your friend's only other problem is that she has mild asthma.

• Design a two-day plan for diet and exercise to help her.

• Explain how you will make sure that the plan does not affect her asthmatic condition.

A2 How do you think a person will feel physically, intellectually, emotionally and socially if they succeed in achieving their plan?

A3 Identify THREE short-term and THREE long-term targets within the plan.

A4 How could the person be supported to keep the plan?

Bill

Bill is 47 years old and believes he is 22 pounds overweight. He smokes 20 cigarettes a day and drinks five bottles of red wine a week. He has discovered that light physical exercise now makes him out of breath, this has worried him. He has turned to you to help him get back to a normal size and weight. He also wants to become fitter. He is 5ft 10 inches tall and weighs 14 stone (he does not use metric measurements).

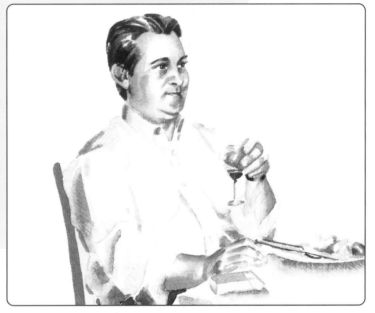

Bill wants to lose weight and get fit

Helping Bill

A1 Convert the measurements in the case study to metric.

A2 Draw up a plan to help Bill stop smoking.

A3 Identify THREE sources of support to help Bill with the plan and explain how each would help.

A4 List THREE short-term and THREE long-term risks to Bill if he continues to smoke.

A5 Present to plan to Bill in a form that he can use.

A6 What are the likely effects on Bill's physical, intellectual, emotional and social well-being after he gives up smoking for six months.

3 Understanding personal development and relationships

Contents

About this unit

You will learn about:

- the stages and patterns of human growth and development
- the different factors that affect human growth and development
- the development of self-concept and personal relationships
- major life changes and how people deal with them
- the role of relationships in personal development.

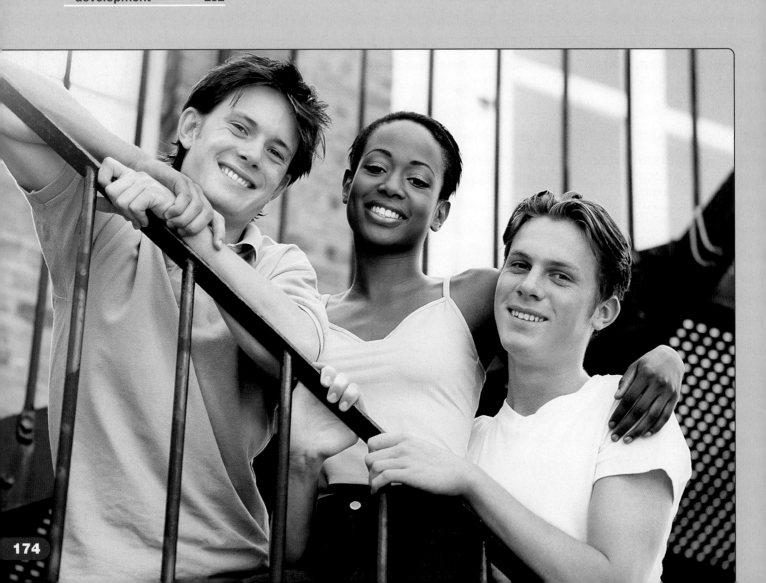

Introducing this unit

We all grow and develop throughout our lives. We develop physically, intellectually, emotionally and socially. When we look at someone, we can tell a lot of things about them from their appearance. We can make a good guess about how old they are. We expect them to be able to do certain things, and to behave in certain ways. For instance:

- we do not expect a six month-old baby to walk

- we do not expect to get good advice about relationships from a five year-old child

- we do not expect a 30 year-old adult to have a tantrum in a supermarket

- we do not expect a 70 year-old adult to be playing football for a premier league team.

When we meet someone who does not behave in the way we expect, we look for a reason.

The reason we can tell so much about people is because nearly all of us develop at a similar rate. Certain changes happen to nearly all of us at about the same time, and this means that we can divide life up into life stages.

Some of these changes happen quite quickly. This means they are very noticeable, for instance a boy's voice breaking, or a girl developing breasts. Others, like ageing, happen very gradually over a long period of time.

A lot of factors influence these changes. This unit will help you understand the changes we experience throughout our lives. It will help you understand what factors influence these changes.

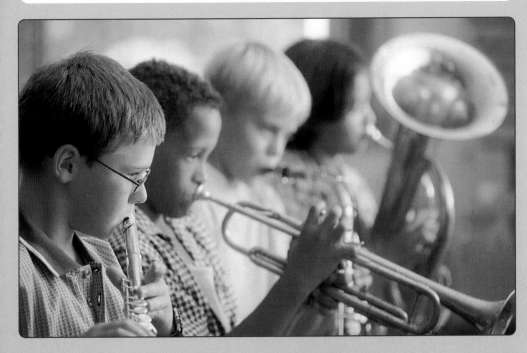

Playing music helps us develop intellectually, emotionally and socially

Human growth and development

Getting started

Individuals grow and develop in a number of ways in each life stage. In this section you will:

- understand what is meant by human growth and development
- understand life stages and when they happen
- understand the patterns of development that take place in each life stage.

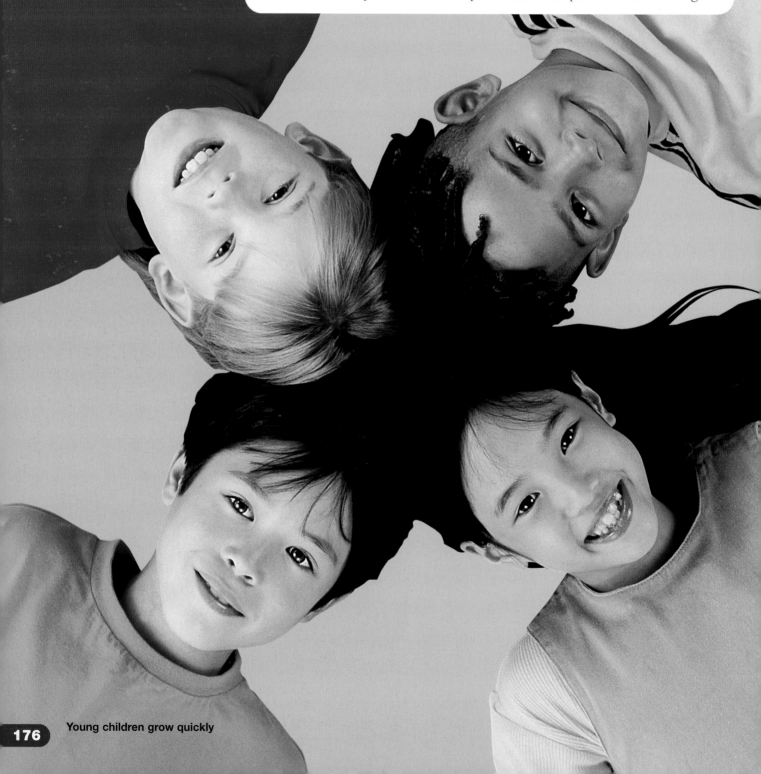

Young children grow quickly

Growth and development

Throughout our lives we grow and develop. We change from being helpless babies who are dependent on their carers to being fully independent adults. When we reach the older adult life stage we may once again, become dependent on others to help meet our needs. The way we change is called human growth and development.

We need to remember that:

- human growth is about increases in physical size, for example, height and weight

- human development is about the way we increase our skills, and develop abilities and emotions.

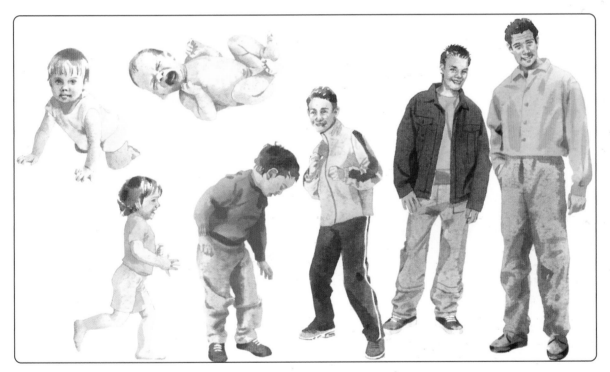

1 What is the difference between 'growth' and 'development'?

Human growth from infancy to adulthood

How we develop

Developmental changes include:

- physical development

- intellectual development

- emotional development

- social development.

You might find it easier to remember these if you think of PIES. Turn back to page 9 to remind yourself what PIES mean.

PIES, see page 9

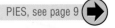 Worksheet 31 – How do individuals grow and develop?
Worksheet 35 – Needs and how they can be met

177

Word check

cognitive – to do with thinking.

Physical development

Physical development is about growth or changes in our bodies. These changes happen to people in each of the different life stages. It is also about how people gain increased control over their bodies and become able to look after themselves and others.

Intellectual development

Intellectual development is about being able to recognise and remember things, and to think about them. Another way of describing this is **cognitive** development. Examples of intellectual development are learning to talk, to read, and to count.

Emotional development

Emotional development is about feelings and how they affect our behaviour. Love, hate, fear, anger, disgust, curiosity, surprise and guilt are all emotions. There are two aspects to emotional development.

- As people **mature**, they experience a wider range of emotions. They get better at understanding the feelings of other people. They develop beliefs about themselves, their self-image and self-esteem.

- Emotional development is also about how a person learns to control their behaviour.

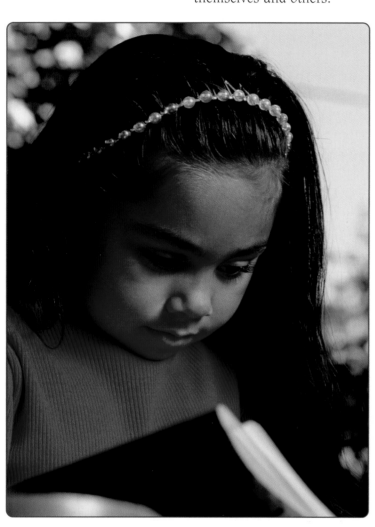

Reading is a way to stimulate our intellectual ability

Word check

mature – when a person's development is complete.

Social development

Social development is about relationships and how a person learns to understand others and develops the skills to get on with them. We learn what other people's expectations of us are in certain situations. This is called socialisation.

 What is the difference between emotional and social development?

Life stages

We can divide a person's life into stages because the same patterns of development usually happen at about the same time in all our lives. Turn back to page 5 to see what these life stages are.

Client groups, see page 5 ➡

3 What are the five life stages?

Infancy (0–3 years)

The table shows some of the physical milestones in an infant's development.

Milestones in physical development

Age	Activity
Three months	• Babies can sit with their head held steady for a few seconds, if supported.
Six months	• Babies have more strength and muscle control. They can lift their head, sit with support and turn their head to look around. • They can pull themselves up when their hands are grasped.
Nine months	• Babies can sit unsupported for ten minutes. • They are starting to move independently by rolling or crawling. • They can pull themselves to stand, and can stand holding on to something for a few moments.
12 months	• Babies can get from a lying to a sitting position without help. • They crawl rapidly. • They can walk by holding on to furniture and stand alone for a few moments.
15 months	• Toddlers can get to their feet alone. • They can walk and crawl upstairs.
18 months	• Infants can run, walk upstairs and crawl downstairs.
Two years	• Infants can walk downstairs.
Three years	• Infants can climb on play equipment, ride a tricycle and throw and catch a ball.

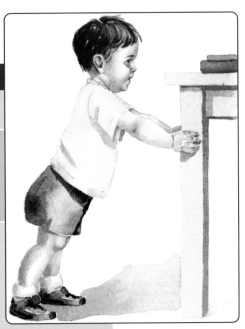

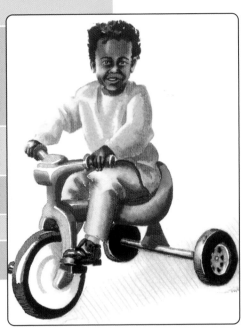

Developing control over our movements can be hard work

Word check

egocentric – only able to see things from your own point of view.

Intellectual development in infancy

At first, infants are **egocentric**. This means they can only see the world from their own point of view. They cannot talk or understand language, so they can only learn through sight, sound, taste, smell and touch. This is why a 6–12 month old baby puts everything in its mouth.

A six month-old child who drops a toy out of their cot will not look for it. If they cannot see it, they do not know that it still exists. By about nine months they learn that objects that they cannot see are still there, and can be retrieved.

As an infant grows, talking and listening become more important ways of learning. They begin to ask questions and put their thoughts into words. Once infants have learned to talk they are always asking 'why' questions. Learning to talk is an important intellectual development in infancy. The table gives some examples of the milestones of intellectual development for an infant.

Milestones in intellectual development

Age	Abilities
Three months	• Babies make noises when they are spoken to.
Nine months	• Babies practise making sounds, repeating syllables like 'mum-mum' and 'dad-dad'. • They begin to learn that the sounds their carers make mean something. • They understand a couple of words, like 'no' and 'bye-bye'.
12 months	• They know their own name and understand several words. • They understand simple commands with gestures, such as 'give it to mummy'.
15 months	• They understand and obey simple commands, for example, 'bring it here'. • They can say a few words and understand many more.
18 months	• They try to join in with nursery rhymes. Soon after this they can put a few words together to make simple sentences.
Two years	• They can use 50 words and understand many more.
Two and a half years	• Infants use 200 words. • They can say a few nursery rhymes. • They ask questions all the time, such as 'what's that?'
Three years	• They have learned a lot more words and can carry on simple conversations with adults.

Emotional development in infancy

Have you ever heard a young baby crying because they are hungry or uncomfortable? If you have, you will know how simple their emotions are. Since they have little control over their bodies, they do not have a wide range of responses to their emotions. As they get older they develop a wider range of emotions. These are connected with other forms of development. For example:

- they have to bond with somebody, and experience **attachment** before they can feel jealous

- they must be able to tell the difference between strangers and people they know before they can feel shy

- if bonding does not occur the child can become disruptive and may feel unloved and unwanted.

Children can experience a wider range of emotions by the time they are two years old. You may have seen a six month-old baby beginning to be shy of strangers. It is common to see a two year-old child showing how jealous they are of a new brother or sister.

At two years old infants still cannot control how they respond to their emotions. You have probably heard mothers talking about the 'terrible twos'. A two year-old will often have tantrums when frustrated. Tantrums are less frequent when infants are three and can control their emotions better.

The way infants are treated by carers affects their developing self-concept. If they are encouraged and treated kindly, they will feel better about themselves than if they are criticised and shouted at. The way they are cared for affects their social development, too.

Social development in infancy

Newborn babies are very interested in faces, and soon get to recognise their main carer. They get to know their carer's face, voice, smell and touch. This is called bonding.

By the time a baby is six weeks old, they smile at their carer. This is a baby's first social action. The baby soon learns to enjoy being played with by people. By the time they are six months old they can tell people they know from strangers. They become shy with people they do not know. They still do not understand that other people have thoughts and feelings. They will not be interested in playing with other children for a long time yet.

- Up to the age of two, infants play alone (solitary play).

- By two years, infants play near other children but do not know how to play with them (parallel play).

- By two and a half years infants are interested by other children playing. They may join in for a few minutes, but still have no idea how to share playthings.

- By the age of three, they play with other children and understand how to share (cooperative play). They can cope with being away from their carer for a few hours.

4 Jack is two years old. Why would he be happier in a parent and toddler group than a playgroup?

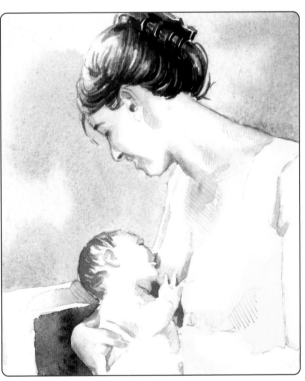

Bonding between mother and baby is important

Danny
CASE STUDY

Danny is one year old. He is achieving the norms for his age. His mother goes out to work one morning each week. While she is at work Danny stays with a childminder. He cried at first when he was left with the childminder, but now he has settled down and is happy.

C1 If Danny is growing and developing to the norm, what physical milestones will he have passed from birth to his present age?

C2 Why do you think Danny cried when he was first left with the childminder? Which aspect of development does this relate to?

C3 How could the childminder help encourage Danny's intellectual development?

Infant growth and development
ACTIVITY

You want to find out about the physical, intellectual and social development of an infant who is around two years of age.

A1 As a group discuss the questions you could ask the child's parents to find out about the child's growth and development.

A2 Produce a short questionnaire that could be used when interviewing the parents about the child's physical, intellectual and social development.

A3 Use the questionnaire to interview the parent(s) about the growth and development of the child.

A4 Assemble all the information you have collected about the child. Draw some conclusions about the infant's growth and development.

Key learning activity

K1 Number the boxes in the table below from 1–4 to show the order in which each developmental milestone normally happens.

Can smile	
Can ride a two-wheeled bike	
Can walk	
Can roll over from front on to back	

K2 Copy the list and by each activity state whether it is a physical, intellectual, emotional or social activity:

- sorting toy bricks into different colours
- playing with toys
- climbing on a climbing frame
- being comforted by mother when crying
- building a tower of bricks.

K3 Give TWO measurements that could be used to assess the growth of infants.

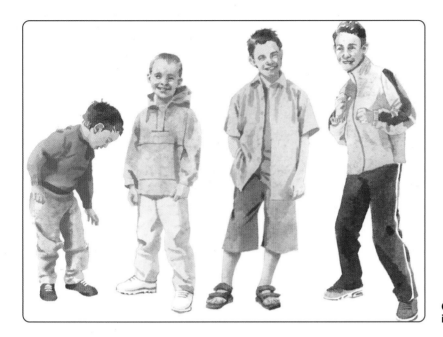

**Growth during childhood
is slower than in infancy**

Childhood

Childhood is the life stage when people develop control over their bodies. Our emotions become more complex as we get older and we have more control over how we respond to them. We develop more communication skills and learn to relate to others.

Physical growth and development in childhood

Physical growth in childhood is more gradual than in infancy, although there is a **growth spurt** between five and seven years.

From five years old children develop their physical skills. They improve their co-ordination and control and can skip, throw and catch accurately, and hit a ball with a bat.

Intellectual development in childhood

During childhood, we learn to talk well. By the end of this stage we understand **concepts**. These are ways in which we use our minds to organise thoughts and information. Think of ways that we group things together in our mind. These are concepts. Concepts include colour, number, size and symbols. A child understands that a number of different red objects are all the same colour, and they know that ten beans is the same number as ten buttons. The child now has a simple understanding of right and wrong.

5 What are concepts?

When a child starts school at around five years old, they begin to learn how to organise their thoughts. They are helped to do this through the various activities provided by the teacher. The child also begins to learn new vocabulary as they listen to other children in their class and the new words introduced by their teacher.

At this stage the child is no longer egocentric. This means that they can now see things from someone else's point of view. They are beginning to be able to work things out, but need to see and touch things to understand and solve problems. They still cannot work things out in their heads by using their imagination.

> **Word check** ✔
>
> **growth spurt** – a rapid period of growth.

> **Word check** ✔
>
> **concept** – the way we organise information in our minds; an abstract idea.

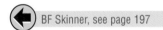
Word check

potential – showing the possibility of achieving to the best of our ability.

What do theorists think about the intellectual development of children? Piaget was a theorist who wrote about child development. This Swiss scientist thought that children were born with some basic abilities and that a person's intellectual **potential** gradually developed as a result of their experiences. Piaget thought that children would try to draw conclusions from their experiences.

Piaget studied the development of children very carefully. He thought that there were several stages in the intellectual development of the child. These were as follows:

- The sensory motor stage that occurs between birth and two years. This is where babies find out about the things around them and what they do.

- The pre-operational stage that occurs between the ages of two and seven years. This is where thought processes are developing. At this stage children need to see and feel things in order to learn.

- The concrete operational stage, which is from seven to 11 years. At this stage of development children can think more logically and follow rules.

Other people who have studied children have different theories about development. These include people such as Skinner (behavourist theories), Bandura (social learning theory) and Erikson (psychoanalytical theories).

◄ BF Skinner, see page 197

6 Can you find out about Bandura's Social learning theory?

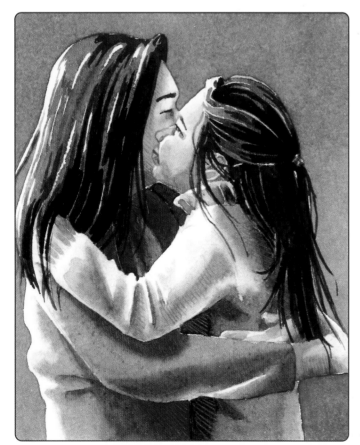

Feeling happy and secure

Emotional development in childhood
Children experience a wider range of emotions than infants.

This is because more complicated emotions depend on other learning and development. For example, it is not possible to feel guilty until we understand the difference between right and wrong.

As children get older they get better at controlling the way they respond to their emotions. They learn that they should express their emotions differently in different situations.

Children still depend on their carers and close family members. How they are treated by their carers is still very important for their self-concept. Now there are other influences as well. As children get older they meet more people outside the family. Their self-concept is affected by their relationships with others – school friends and teachers, for example. If they are popular in school, and have lots of friends, it will have a positive effect on their self-concept. Being unpopular, or bullied can have a negative effect.

For example, a child who has a positive self-concept will feel secure and will probably be full of energy and enthusiasm about the things he or she is asked to do. On the other hand, a child who is bullied is likely to have a negative self-image. They may become withdrawn or they could also become aggressive and bully other children.

Having emotional **stability** is important in the development of the child as it is likely to influence their actions and attitudes throughout their lives.

Word check ✓

stability – things not changing, remaining the same.

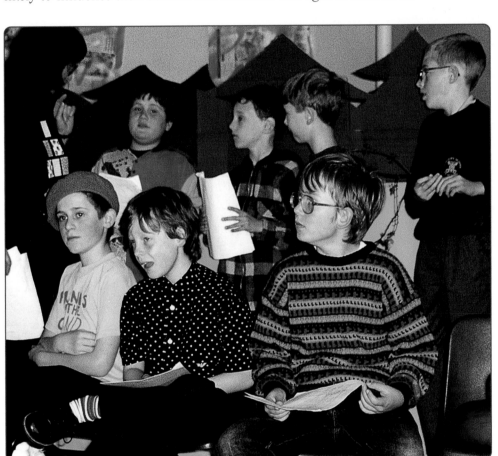

Enjoying school, rehearsing a play

Social development in childhood

By the age of four, children need other children to play with. They are much better at understanding the feelings of others. They understand how to take turns. They can be separated from their main carer without distress.

By five years old children are attending school, meeting lots of new children and choosing their own friends. They cooperate with other children in games, and understand rules and fairness. Because children understand more about how others are feeling, it becomes more important for them to have the approval of the other children.

By the age of seven years children are aware of sexual differences and prefer to play with children of the same sex. This will continue until adolescence.

7 James is four years old and about to start primary school. How has his personal development prepared him for this?

Jessica
CASE STUDY

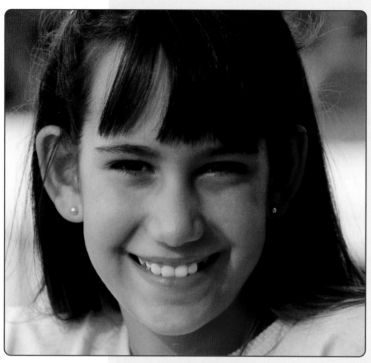

Jessica aged 8

Jessica is eight years old. She has grown quite a bit over the last two years. She likes looking at herself in the mirror. She thinks she looks like her mum.

She enjoys going to school as she likes learning new things. She has started to learn French and she is quite good at the subject. She also likes playing with her friends in the playground.

She goes with her friends to junior youth club on Friday evenings. They enjoy the activities of cooking and orienteering, although they can do lots of different things.

C1 How might attending junior youth club help Jessica's intellectual and social development?

C2 Describe Jessica's emotional development during this life stage.

C3 How might learning French help Jessica's development?

C4 Why is 'emotional stability' important for a child?

C5 Carry out some research to find out what Erikson thought about Jessica's stage of development.

C6 Compare Piaget's view of development with that of Erikson.

Key learning activity
ACTIVITY

K1 Identify THREE physical changes that occur in childhood.

K2 Describe how going to school could help Jessica's intellectual and social development.

K3 Here is a list of activities that people in the childhood life stage are able to do. For each write down whether it is a physical, intellectual or social activity:

- learning a language
- playing rounders
- feeling pleased for getting a question right in class
- discussing things with friends
- going skateboarding.

Adolescence (11 – 18 years)

Adolescence is the life stage in which a people achieve sexual maturity. They also develop the intellectual skills to think in an abstract way. Adolescents start to become independent and develop a sense of their personal identity.

Physical growth and development in adolescence

Both boys and girls have a growth spurt caused by the production of **hormones**. A boy's growth spurt is usually greater than a girl's. This is why adult men are usually taller and heavier than women. The most important physical development in adolescence is **puberty**, when adolescents become sexually mature. Girls can experience puberty from the age of 11. Boys may experience puberty slightly later.

What causes the changes in adolescence?
The hormones that produce the growth spurt in adolescence also cause the sex organs to produce **sex hormones**.

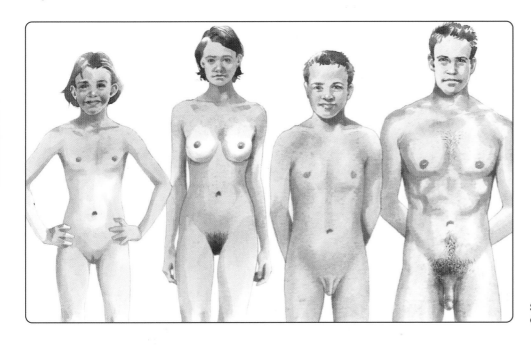

Secondary sexual characteristics

> **Word check** ✓
>
> **hormone** – chemical messenger that affects the way our bodies function.
> **puberty** – the physical features of becoming sexually mature.

> **Word check** ✓
>
> **sex hormone** – chemical messenger in the body that affect our sexual development and activities.

Changes that take place in adolescence

Physical development in girls	Physical development in boys
• develop breasts	• penis and testes grow larger
• grow pubic and underarm hair	• grow pubic, facial and underarm hair
• hips widen	• muscles develop; chest and shoulders broaden
• start to menstruate (have periods)	• may have wet dreams, which shows they can ejaculate sperm
	• larnyx (voice box) grows, voice breaks and becomes deeper

Intellectual development in adolescence

Adolescence is a time when there are rapid changes in the mind as well as in the body. It is a time when the adolescent learns to think in different ways. They can understand more difficult concepts than children. They learn to synthesise information – to blend information together from several different sources. They can also use their imagination to solve problems in their heads, without having to see them.

Sometimes this new ability to think for themselves leads to arguments between adolescents and their parents and disagreements with others. Adolescents want to exercise their intellectual ability to make their own decisions. Within a **peer group** someone who has developed the ability to think independently can exercise power over other members of the group.

Emotional development in adolescence

The hormone changes responsible for puberty also affect adolescents' emotions. They have mood swings. They may be excited one minute and depressed the next. They may be very moody and get angry very easily. It is sometimes very difficult for adolescents and their families to cope with these mood swings.

At the same time, adolescents are looking for a sense of personal identity, or to discover 'who' they are. One way they do this is by reacting against their parents' ideas and values. These may be ideas about politics or religion, or smoking and drinking.

Insecurity can be a part of adolescent emotional development, so parents and friends need to be very patient and understanding. Adolescence is a time when our **personality** is developed, based on our individual characteristics, habits and experiences.

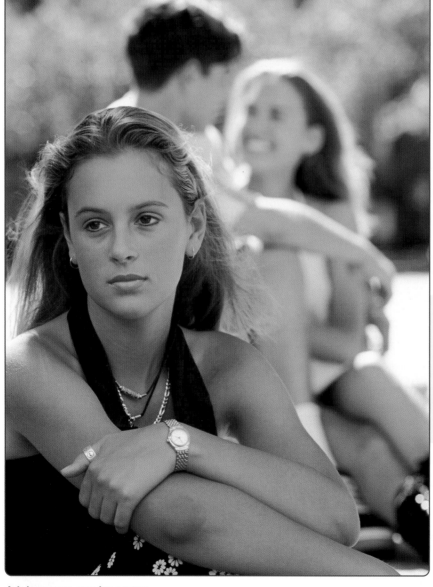

Adolescence can be a very difficult time

Social development in adolescence

Adolescents need to develop independence from their parents. Their parents' opinions become less important to them than the opinions of other adolescents. It becomes very important to fit in with their peer group and gain their approval. It may be important to wear the right kind of clothes, or listen to the right kind of music to fit in with a group.

In early adolescence teenagers tend to do things together in groups. It is in group situations that experimental behaviour takes place, for example, trying alcohol or drugs.

With increasing sexual maturity, adolescents begin to look for a partner of the opposite sex. They may start to experiment with sexual relationships.

8 Why do many adolescents frequently argue with their parents?

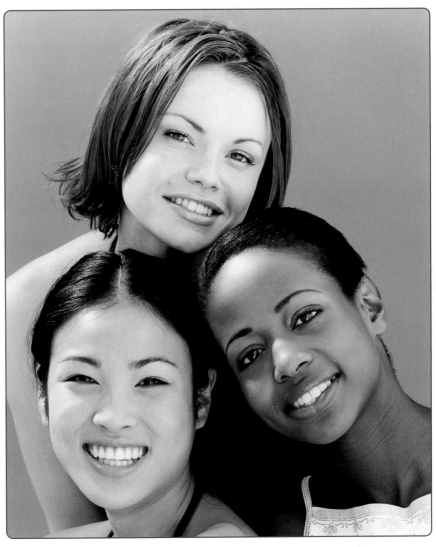

Adolescence is a time for both making and breaking friendships

Marcus

CASE STUDY

Marcus is 15 years old. He likes being in a group of people of his own age. When he is with his friends he likes to take the lead. He is very quick thinking and likes to have a joke. His friends usually follow his suggestions. Marcus does not get on with his parents very well. His social life often means that he does not get home until one or two o'clock in the morning. His parents are not very impressed with this. They want him to do well at school and go on to college.

C1 Why do you think Marcus likes to be the group leader?

C2 How could Marcus's parents help to improve their relationship their son?

C3 Describe the physical development of an adolescent.

C4 How do feelings of insecurity affect the emotional development of adolescents?

Key learning activities

ACTIVITY

K1 Identify FOUR characteristics of physical development during adolescence.

K2 Describe THREE social changes that occur during adolescence.

K3 Describe the changes that are taking place between Marcus and his parents. Explain why the changes are happening.

Adulthood

Adulthood is the period when the individual has achieved physical maturity. Compulsory education has finished and the young adult either tries to find work or goes on to further or higher education studies. Settling into a career becomes a very important part of adult life . Most people find a partner, leave home and start their own families.

Physical growth and development in adulthood

Adults are fully mature and there is little growth during adulthood. Adults tend to gain weight as they age, but this is probably due more to a **sedentary** lifestyle than the ageing process.

Physical development is completed early in adulthood. Physical decline starts quite early, although at first it is too gradual to notice. An important physical development for women towards the end of this life stage is the **menopause**. Usually between the ages of 45 and 55, women's periods stop, and they are no longer able to have children. This is caused by hormonal changes in the body.

Sometimes a woman may feel a sense of loss when the menopause occurs. Others will be glad that they no longer have to worry about becoming pregnant and so have a sense of freedom.

Intellectual development in adulthood

Intellectual development continues throughout adulthood. Getting a job involves learning new skills. If a person wants to progress in a career, these skills have to be developed and extended. Most people will have more than one job during their lives. This is because people learn or develop new skills and may want to apply these in new situations. Also, new jobs are created that need different skills. We now talk about 'lifelong learning' for people to update their skills and learn new ones.

Even outside the workplace, adulthood is a period of intellectual development. Many skills are needed when a person leaves home and lives independently. These include cooking and managing a home and a budget. All of these have to be learned. Raising children involves learning new skills.

As adults age, they react more slowly and find it more difficult to remember things under pressure. However, to balance this, they have learned from experience and are better at solving problems and making decisions. This compensates for any decline in intellectual ability over the life stage.

Word check

sedentary – inactive; not getting very much exercise.

Word check ✓

menopause – the end of a woman's reproductive life.

Emotional development in adulthood

When we talk about someone behaving in a mature manner, we usually mean that they are controlling the way they respond to the emotions that they are feeling.

When we leave home, we have to be independent and self-reliant to cope. Living with a long-term partner takes a high level of emotional maturity if the relationship is not to break down when there are problems. People have to understand their own emotions and those of their partner. They also have to be able to control the way they respond to their emotions. If they cannot do this, it can result in the breakdown of the relationship. It can lead to violence if one partner cannot control emotions such as jealousy and anger.

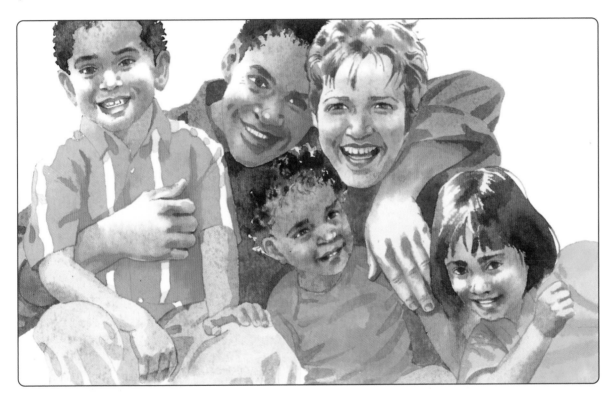

Having children means more responsibility

The arrival of children means accepting new responsibilities. Babies are very demanding. This can cause a lot of stress to the people who care for them. Adults have to be emotionally mature to cope.

- If adults are not able to put the needs of the baby before their own, then the baby may be neglected.

- If they cannot control emotions such as anger, then the child may be abused.

- If one partner is immature and jealous of the attention given to the baby, then the parents' relationship may break down.

The jobs that adults do are an important part of their identity and self-concept. This means that a job has an emotional aspect. A person may feel proud of their job, and think that they have been successful in getting it. They may be dissatisfied with their job and feel that they could do better. Someone who does not have a job may feel a failure. "What do you do?" is often one of the first things we ask when we meet someone new.

Social development in adulthood

When young adults leave home, they have to develop new types of relationship. They may have a partner or get married and this means making decisions, accepting responsibility and sharing. Relationships with parents change. Young adults start to relate to their parents more as equals. Parents realise that their offspring now take responsibility for themselves and maybe others as well.

Starting a job involves developing working relationships with people. These are a different type of relationship. You do not have the same choice about working relationships as you do with social relationships. We sometimes distinguish them by calling them **formal** and **informal relationships**. Working relationships are formal because there are rules to be followed. You know that some people at work can tell you what to do.

9 How does getting a job contribute towards an individual's personal development?

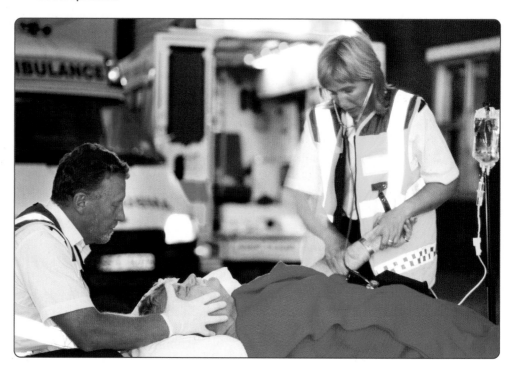

Adults learn to accept responsibility

10 How are working relationships different from social relationships?

Settling down with a long-term partner can bring changes to people's social lives. They may mix more with other couples. With marriage comes a set of new relatives, or in-laws. Even if people are just living together, this often involves building new relationships with their partner's family.

11 How might the arrival of their first child change the relationship between a couple?

As adults near the older adult life stage, they may find that their parents are declining physically, and may begin to depend on them. This brings increased responsibility.

Word check

formal relationship – relationship, such as a working relationship, that has rules about how people should behave.

Word check

informal relationship – casual or social relationship.

Later adulthood (65+ years)

This life stage starts with retirement from work. An older adult has to get used to the idea that they are no longer a wage earner. They are not usually responsible for others. This new role can cause some people to feel upset if they have not prepared for retirement.

Physical growth and development in later adulthood

People become shorter in late adulthood as their posture becomes less upright and their spine becomes compressed. A person can lose up to 7cm in height!

The physical decline that started in early adulthood becomes more obvious, especially after the age of 75 years.

These are some of the expected physical changes:

- skin wrinkles because of loss of elastic tissues

- hair thins and goes grey; men often have hair loss.

- bones are more fragile as thinning makes them lighter and more brittle, particularly in women

- body organs are less efficient, including the heart, lungs, kidneys and liver

- sight worsens as the eye's lens stiffens and is less able to focus on close objects, making reading difficult. The retina becomes less sensitive to light, and an older person may need a brighter light

- hearing deteriorates with the gradual deterioration of the mechanism of the ear

- mobility may be affected as joints stiffen and become worn or inflamed.

A number of things are affected by a deteriorating nervous system:

- sense of taste and smell is reduced

- older people are less sensitive to cold, making them more at risk from hypothermia

- balance is often poor, and falls more likely.

Many of these problems can be overcome or managed so that the older adult can enjoy a better quality of life.

Keeping fit can help to maintain our health and well-being and may help to prevent or delay some aspects of physical decline. Activities such as swimming, walking and jogging can all help to maintain our health and mobility.

Spectacles and hearing aids can compensate for deteriorating sight and hearing. If joints become damaged, particularly hips and knees, they can be replaced. These operations are now common and are not the major events they were a few years ago.

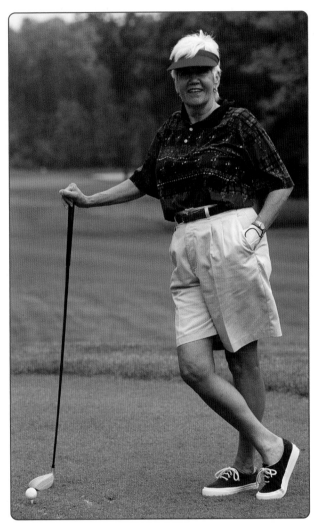

Keeping active can help maintain health and well-being

Hypothermia, see page 162

193

Intellectual development in later adulthood

Because of the gradual deterioration of the nervous system, older people have difficulty in remembering things quickly, particularly when they are under pressure. Their reaction times are also slower.

However, they may have more experience and judgement than a younger person. They may make better decisions as a result.

Some older people become too confused to manage their own affairs. Confusion is different from dementia. With dementia actual brain cells stop functioning. This is permanent. Confusion is temporary and usually passes when the person is less flustered.

Social development in later adulthood

Later adulthood is a time of great social change for most people.

The official retirement age for men is 65. Soon men and women will retire at the same age. As lifespan increases and people become increasingly healthy and active in later adulthood, they will spend a larger part of their lives in retirement, unless the retirement age is raised.

Some older people miss regular contact with workmates. Others enjoy having more time to spend on their hobbies and interests. How people are affected may depend on their income. Many older people with pensions from jobs are well off. Others who do not have a good occupational pension may find it hard to make ends meet. Some older adults use their retirement to travel around the world or to start new activities.

The children of older adults will probably be adult, living their own lives. They may live some distance away from their parents. The older adult may feel that they are not needed and could feel isolated. On the other hand, there may be the pleasures of grandchildren, without being responsible for them.

As people get older, they suffer more **bereavements** – of friends, close relatives, and perhaps their partner. They have to adapt to a smaller social circle.

> **Word check** ✓
>
> **bereavement** – losing someone close to you or well known to you.

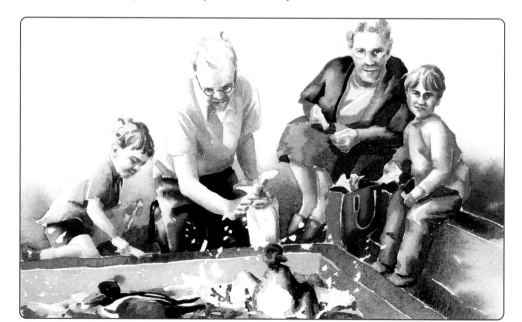

Being with grandparents can be fun

Mr Davies and his family CASE STUDY

Mr Davies is 70 years old and lives with his wife in their own home. He has a good pension from his job, and considers himself quite well off. Their two children are married and live nearby. They have five grandchildren that they see regularly.

Mr Davies drives, but he is thinking of giving up his car. Mr Davies took up painting when he retired, and enjoys doing this now he has given up hillwalking. He is a member of a number of local organisations. Mr Davies sometimes says he does not know how he found time to go to work.

C1 Explain why painting is a better hobby for Mr Davies than hillwalking.

C2 Why do you think Mr Davies is considering giving up his car?

C3 Describe the social developments for Mr and Mrs Davies in the life stage they are in.

C4 How does an individual's relationship with their child change throughout their lifespan?

Key learning activity ACTIVITY

K1 Describe FOUR physical changes that occur in older adults.

K2 How is an older adult's emotional development likely to be affected in this life stage?

K3 Identify TWO intellectual responsibilities and TWO social responsibilities that occur in the older adult life stage.

K4 Explain how being a member of voluntary community organisations can contribute to Mr Davies' intellectual and social health and well-being.

Factors that affect growth and development

Getting started

What factors affect human growth and development?

How can factors influence an individual's health, well-being and life opportunities?

Physical, social, emotional, economic and environmental factors all influence people's growth and development.

In this section you will:

- find out about the factors that affect the way people grow and develop
- look at how the different factors affect people's growth and development
- understand how these factors affect people's health, well-being and life opportunities.

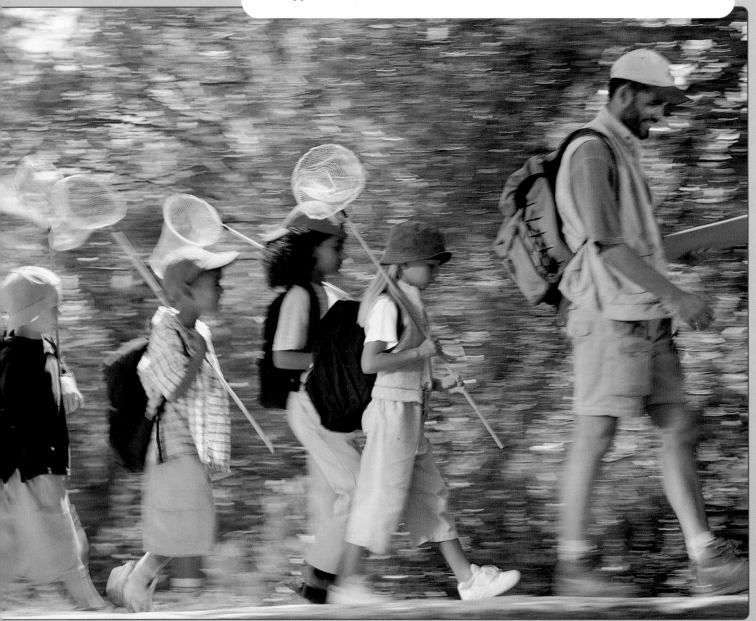

Making good use of our leisure time helps our growth and development

Growth and development are affected by a number of different factors. These include:

- physical factors
- economic factors
- social and emotional factors
- environmental factors.

Physical factors

Physical factors include genetic inheritance, diet, the amount and type of physical activity we undertake and any illnesses and diseases.

Genetic inheritance

Genes are found in every cell of our bodies. They control our characteristics. Turn back to pages 125–129 to remind yourself about genes and how they influence our development.

Genes, see page 125

Some genes cause diseases that affect the way that people develop. **Genetic disorders** cause a variety of diseases and other problems. They can cause physical and learning disabilities. Sometimes they result in early death. Some of these genetic disorders can be **hereditary**. An example of an hereditary genetic disorder is haemophilia which affects the blood.

⑫ Find out what support groups are available to help people with hereditary or genetic diseases.

Word check

genetic disorder – disease or problem caused by our genes.

hereditary – characteristics passed from our parents.

Nature v nurture

We sometimes talk about **nature** and **nurture**. By nature, we mean the genetic influences on our development. Nurture is about all the other influences. These are often called **environmental** factors. They are the things around us that have an influence on us. Family, education and where we live are examples of environmental factors.

How can environmental factors influence our development?

Our environment can have a major effect on our development. For example, if we live in an area where the crime rate is high we may be afraid to go out in case we are mugged. Our personal development would be affected. We may always want to have someone with us when we go out. We might be afraid to go out when it is dark. People who are scared like this can become socially isolated and afraid.

Word check

nature – the qualities we are born with that make us what we are.

nurture – how we are influenced when we are young by the environment around us, including other people.

environmental – to do with our surroundings.

Theorists such as John B Watson have argued that environmental influences are those that have the greater impact on the development of our personality, rather than hereditary (inborn) factors.

The question is this: is how we behave born in us or is it learnt?

BF Skinner and others have studied behaviour and have concluded that our learning is shaped by our direct personal experiences. Skinner thinks that this is likely to mean that we will want to repeat any good experiences we have and that we will want to avoid any that we have not enjoyed. Skinner called the things we would want to repeat 'positive reinforcements'. Examples of different types of positive reinforcements are food, praise and money. This theory is known as **behaviourist theory**. It means that we learn from 'trial and error'. We learn from our experiences, the things in our environment that influence us.

Word check

behaviourist theory – the theory that people learn the ways of behaving through rewards and punishments.

Many people consider that our development is influenced by both nature (the qualities we are born with) and nurture (how we are influenced when we are young by the environment and people around us). It is most likely that the combination of nature and nurture influence a person's individual health and well-being and life opportunities.

13 What is meant by the nature–nurture debate?

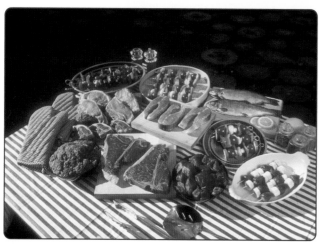

We are what we eat

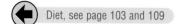

Diet, see page 103 and 109

The effect of diet on development

Eating can be a social activity as well as contributing to our physical health and well-being. A family may enjoy breakfast together. Or, if people are leaving for school and work they may all meet together for an evening meal.

How the food we eat influences our development

Diet is an important influence on growth and development. The food we eat meets our physical needs. Turn back to pages 103–108 to find out the sources of these foods and their function in the body.

It is important that we make sure we have a balanced diet. Turn back to pages 109–112 and then answer the question.

14 What is a balanced diet?

What we need for a balanced diet depends upon:

• our age

• our size

• our gender

• the amount of exercise we take

• factors such as pregnancy and breastfeeding.

If we do not have a balanced diet, our growth and development can be seriously affected.

Diet in infancy
Breast milk or infant formula (powdered milk) contains everything a young baby needs for a balanced diet. If they do not get the nutrients they need their growth and development maybe affected. For example, they may not grow at the rate expected for their age.

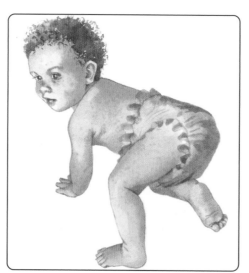

In later infancy more energy-giving foods are required

After the age of six months babies are more active, so they use more energy. Parents will start giving their baby solid foods. This is called **weaning**. If babies are fed too much carbohydrate and fat at this stage, they may become overweight. This makes it much more difficult for them to stand and walk. In later infancy children become more active and continue to grow rapidly.

15 Why is it important for an infant to have the correct nutrients in the right proportions?

Diet in childhood

If children get more energy from fats and sugars than they use, it is likely that they will put on weight and this could lead to the risk of becoming obese. Children who are overweight or obese are often teased by their peers and this can lead to emotional problems. In extreme cases this can lead to school phobia (staying away from school), and so the child's education can be affected. Diet, combined with other factors, can have a very strong influence on the development of children.

Children often like to eat fast foods such as burgers and chips. If they eat too much of this type of food it can lead to mobility problems. As they become overweight they are not easily able to join in activities such as sport or dancing. Being fat also affects the child's self-esteem. They are likely to have a low opinion of themselves and may dislike their appearance. This may cause them to become isolated and withdrawn from friends and family.

Diet in adolescence

Adolescents often need energy foods and protein because they have a growth spurt. Most of this energy should come from carbohydrates.

Girls in this life stage are often very aware of what they eat. This is because they want to have a good figure and look attractive. Girls sometimes diet to help lose weight.

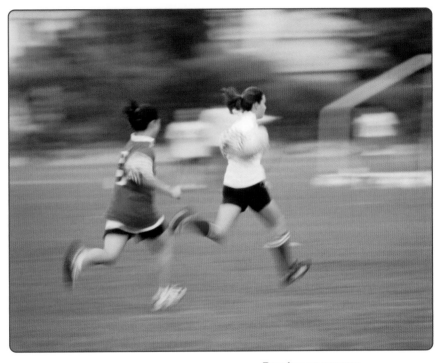

Burning up energy

There are two eating disorders called **anorexia** and **bulimia**. Anorexia is where people, usually girls, stop eating because they 'see themselves' as being fat. Most girls who suffer from anorexia are not fat, but they think of themselves as being fat. When they look in the mirror they do not see their true image but a fatter, less attractive image. People who have bulima eat and then make themselves sick or take laxatives. This prevents the body from absorbing the nutrients it needs.

Both illnesses can affect the development of the adolescent and can cause bowel disorders and other conditions that can affect them throughout their lifespan.

Word check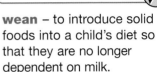

wean – to introduce solid foods into a child's diet so that they are no longer dependent on milk.

Word check ✓

anorexia – illness where the sufferer does not eat to avoid putting on weight.

Word check ✓

bulimia – disorder where people make themselves vomit in order to keep their weight down.

Diet in adulthood

Not all adults have the same dietary needs. An athlete or somebody who has a hard manual job needs much more energy than somebody who works in an office.

Pregnant women need more of some nutrients for their growing babies. If they do not get them, the baby will take what it needs and leave the mother short of nutrients.

 Diet, see pages 109-112

16 Mr Roberts works as a builder. His partner is six months pregnant and works in an office. How do their nutritional needs differ? (Look back at Unit 2 to help you answer this question.)

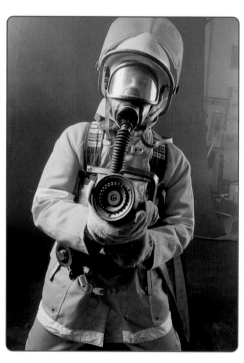

A firefighter on duty uses a lot of energy

If we eat a well-balanced diet, and have regular eating patterns, we are more likely to be healthy. If we eat excessively or have an unbalanced diet we are more likely to develop conditions and illnesses that affect our development.

In the UK people have become more experimental in their choice of meals. More people get a curry or a Chinese takeaway, for example, than they used to. Diet is often linked to social activity. We may go out for a meal with friends or invite them to our own home for a meal. We may have a barbecue and ask friends round. These are social occasions where we can enjoy eating and sharing with others. Having a choice of food and eating it in pleasant surroundings is likely to help us to be happy and contented. It contributes to our emotional well-being.

17 How is diet linked to social activity?

It is unusual for one diet-related factor to cause major health problems. However, when poor diet is combined with other factors such as stress or poor living conditions, then ill-health is likely to result.

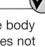

Diet in late adulthood

It is important that older people (over 65 years) have enough energy foods to enable them to maintain their body temperature. Older people are also more at risk of **dehydration** through not drinking enough water. Because the ageing process means that the kidneys are less efficient, older people normally have to go to the toilet more often. Sometimes getting to the toilet is difficult because of mobility problems. They may be tempted to drink less to avoid this, and there is a danger that they will not get enough water for their bodies to work properly.

Word check ✓

dehydration – the body loses water and does not have enough to work properly.

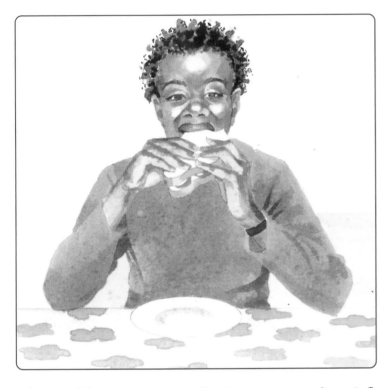

Lack of hot meals can affect health and well-being.

Whatever life stage we are in diet is important and can influence our development.

The effect of physical activity on development

Physical activity can be any type of exercise or recreational activity. Walking to the shops or mowing the lawn are both forms of physical activity. Physical activity can help meet our emotional and social needs as well. Turn back to pages 113–117 to remind yourself all about exercise, its importance and the different types of physical activities that we can do to help maintain health and well-being.

Exercise, see page 113

We need to take part in physical activity throughout our lives. The type of exercise that is right for us depends on our stage of physical development.

Exercise and recreation have emotional and social effects through:

- reducing stress
- relieving depression
- improving self-esteem.

Many children get enough physical activity by walking to school, and playing games. However, there are worries that some children may not get enough physical activity. As a result, more children are becoming unfit and obese. There could be several reasons for this.

- More parents have cars and drive their children to school instead of letting them walk or cycle. They may do this because of worries about the danger of traffic or the risk of abduction. It may also be because more parents work, and do not have the time to walk to school with their children.

- Children and adolescents may be more interested in watching television and playing computer games, leaving less time for physical activities.

- The demands of the national curriculum can mean there is less time available during the school day for activities such as swimming and other sports.

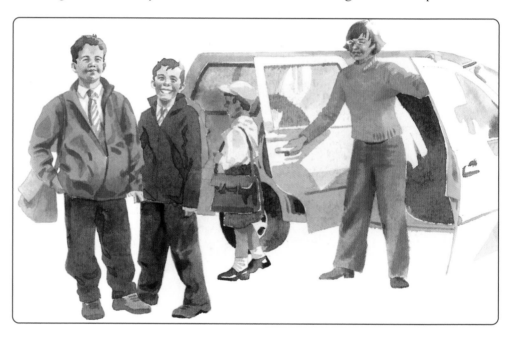

Who walks?

Fewer people work in jobs that need physical effort. Many more people now work in office jobs. Some jobs are physically easier because most of the work is done by machinery. This means that most types of work do not provide the amount of physical activity that is needed to keep healthy.

Adults can make sure that they get some physical activity by doing housework or gardening and walking to the shops. If they do not do many of these things, they have to take care that they get sufficient exercise, perhaps by playing team sports, running or going to the gym.

For older people physical activity may be painful because of rheumatism or arthritis, but they do need exercise, just as in any other life stage. They may need specially organised exercise programmes that are within their physical abilities.

The effect of illness and disease on growth and development

Some illnesses have short-term physical effects. We can have diarrhoea and sickness. We may ache all over or have spots. There are other illnesses that have longer term, more serious effects. It can take a long time to recover from glandular fever, for example.

Illness and disease can be linked to our diet. Lack of iron in our diet can cause tiredness. Harmful bacteria in our food can cause food poisoning. During our lifetime we will all experience illness and disease.

Childhood illnesses

Most illnesses affect an infant's physical development just for a short while. The infant usually makes up for any loss in growth and development when they recover. However, some common childhood illnesses can have long-term effects and serious developmental consequences, sometimes leading to death. Turn back to pages 125–128 to remind yourself about genetic diseases.

Genetics, see page 125

Vaccinations can help prevent us getting some diseases, such as meningitis, whooping cough and tuberculosis. One vaccine that you may have heard of is the MMR vaccine. This single vaccination given to young children can prevent measles, mumps and rubella.

Physical illness and disease can affect our emotional, intellectual and social development. For example, if a child misses a lot of school, they miss learning opportunities as well as mixing and socialising with other children.

Illness in adult life

Serious illness in adulthood may mean that someone cannot work, so they lose the social contact. This may also have emotional effects. People may have depression and lowered self-esteem if they are unable to work.

In late adulthood many people have **degenerative** illnesses such as arthritis and rheumatism. These have the physical effect of making it difficult for them to care for themselves. Other illnesses, such as Alzheimer's disease, have intellectual effects, such as confusion and memory loss. Having to rely on others for everyday care tasks may have emotional effects. People who are unable to care for themselves may become depressed. This is likely to happen if their carers are not careful to offer them choices. If illness makes people less mobile, they may find it difficult to leave their homes. This will have social effects and they may become isolated.

You should remember that:

- happy and contented people are less likely to be ill

- a balanced diet can contribute to good health

- physical activity can contribute to the absence of illness and disease.

> **Word check**
>
> **degenerative** – where an organ, or body process slowly begins to break down or stop functioning.

Belinda

Belinda is an identical twin. She is very close to her sister. They both have fair hair and blue eyes. When they were children they had the usual childhood illnesses but Belinda also developed a mild form of meningitis and was away from school for several weeks.

At school they both did quite well in their examinations but Belinda found the language classes quite difficult. When she was ill she missed quite a few lessons and found it hard to catch up.

Both Belinda and her sister like playing the piano and enjoy cross-country running. When they were younger they used to go running with their father at the weekends. He was a member of the county cross-country running club. Their father taught them how to use a computer when they were six years old.

Belinda has a job as a computer programmer. Her sister also works with computers but in an office at the other end of the town. They meet for lunch twice a week and each brings a friend with them. They usually have a light lunch of jacket potato and salad.

On Thursdays they play badminton in a group of four and on Saturdays they go swimming. They are members of the swimming club.

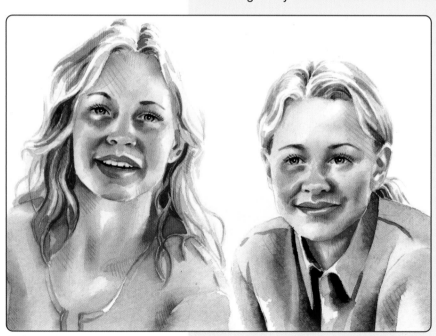

Belinda is an identical twin

C1 Belinda's growth and development has been influenced by several factors. List SIX factors that have influenced her development and give an example of each.

C2 Explain how Belinda's family has influenced her development.

C3 Using the case study for Belinda discuss the nature v nurture features. Give examples to illustrate the points you are making.

C4 Think of your own development or find out about the development of a friend. Describe FOUR factors that have influenced either your own or their personal development. Give examples for each.

Key learning activity

K1 List THREE physical factors that could influence a person's development.

K2 Describe how illness and disease could affect a person's development.

K3 Explain how physical activity has been a factor that has affected Belinda's growth and development.

Social and emotional factors

Social and emotional factors that can affect development include:

- gender
- family relationships
- friendships
- educational experiences
- employment and unemployment
- ethnicity and religion
- life experiences including birth, marriage, divorce and death.

The effect of gender on growth and development

Gender is not the same as sex. An individual's sex depends on their genes. Gender is about the way society expects people of each sex to behave. In other words, gender affects an individual's life opportunities because some jobs, sports or activities will be seen as being appropriate for males and others for females.

It is difficult for people to be themselves if everybody around expects them to behave in certain ways according to their gender. For example, a boy may be given a train and a girl a doll. The child has no choice about some of the toys they are given.

Since part of their intellectual and social development happens through play, their development can be affected. They may start to think that dolls are only for girls to play with and trains are specially for boys. This is known as stereotyping.

At school, children were once told that some activities were suitable for girls, for example, hockey and netball, and some were suitable for boys, for example, football and cricket. A girl who wanted to play football found it difficult to be accepted. Similarly, boys were expected to be better at science, and girls at languages. Although this should not happen now, without meaning to, people can still encourage boys and girls to choose particular subjects based on a gender bias. This will affect personal development as they may find themselves studying a subject that is not the one in which they can achieve the best results.

Stereotyping

The effect of gender on employment opportunities

There are laws against discrimination in employment on the grounds of gender. Some people still believe that some jobs are more suitable for men and some for women. At one time, nearly all doctors were men, and nearly all nurses were women. This is now changing and there are a lot of women doctors and male nurses. The caring profession was once seen as a women's job, but more men are entering it. Many people are still put off applying for jobs if they see them as not appropriate for their gender.

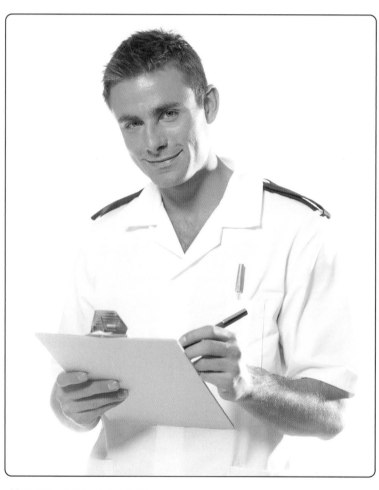

Men are now entering jobs in the care sector

The effect of family relationships on growth and development

Families are very important and can be a major influence on life opportunities. A child's social class depends on their parents. The class we are in can influence the opportunities that we have.

An adult's social class is often based on **economic** factors and the job they do. For example, according to the table on page 147, a GP is considered to be in a higher social class than a lorry driver.

Our economic status can affect our opportunities. Doctors, for example, may encourage their children to stay on at school and succeed in their education. A GP has had first-hand experience of higher education and knows the benefits it can bring.

Someone who left school at 16 might not expect their own children to stay on at school or college. They may not be able to afford to help their children through university. Our social class can have an influence on our growth and development.

Our position in the family can influence our development. If we are the youngest, brothers and sisters might protect us from others. Or on the other hand we could be blamed for everything they do wrong!

18 How does our position in the family affect our development?

The views and opinions that we hear in our own family when we are talking together may also influence our growth and development. Many people adopt their family's views and opinions on subjects such as politics, religion, punishment, law and order and how services should be run. We may hear these views many times within our homes and may agree with them. Some people support the same football team because other members of the family are fans. In other words we often follow family tradition.

The effect of friendships on growth and development

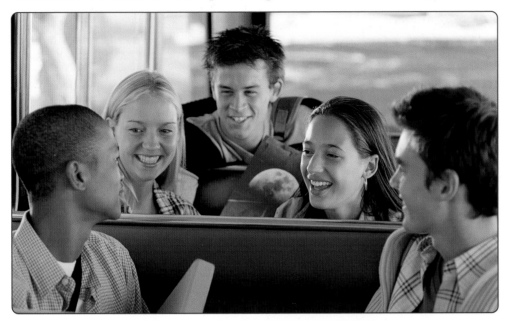

Friends

Friendships are important to growth and development in all life stages. Most people have some close friends that they share personal things with. Then there are other friends that share the same interests. Our friends give us emotional and social support, they:

- listen when we have a problem

- share our good times

- share our activities and interests.

Hopefully we are there when they need us as well!

Sometimes friends can be a bad influence. We may do things that we know are wrong because we do not want to let our friends down. We are 'led' by our friends. Our friends might want us to stay away from school or encourage us to get drunk. Our friends influence us because we do not want to be 'different' and want to keep their friendship. Sometimes it is very hard to say 'no' to them.

Our friends can influence our development positively or negatively. Whether our friends influence us in a good or bad way, we should remember that anything that results from our actions can influence our growth and development. For example, if one teenager persuaded another to go shoplifting on a regular basis, they may be caught. One possible effect on their development could be that they might be sent to a young offenders' institution. The effect on their development could be that they would lose their freedom. They would be taken away from their families and could lose their jobs and friends.

19 How can friends have a negative affect on our development?

Most of our friends have a positive effect on our development.

Brendan and Jim

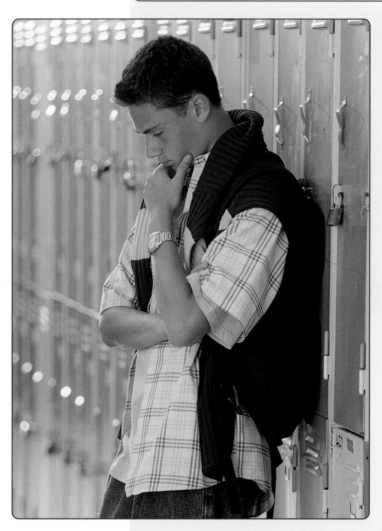

Brendan does not want his mates to see that he is upset

Brendan is 15. He has been going out with Kim for three months. He is very happy and looks forward to their dates. A friend of Kim's hands Brendan a note during the lunch break at school. Brendan reads the note. Kim does not want to go out with him any more.

Brendan just wants to cry, but cannot because he is in school and he does not want his mates to see he is upset. Jim, Brendan's friend, notices the note and guesses what has happened. He goes over to Brendan and asks him if Brendan will go with him down to the local shop.

Jim asks Brendan what the matter is. Brendan tells him and they talk about what has happened. Jim suggests that they meet that evening to talk some more. He also offers to talk to Kim to find out what the problem is.

This is an example of a positive effect on development because of a friendship. Jim saw that his friend was upset. He provided support and a chance for Brendan to talk about his problems. He did not want his friend to be alone that evening so he offered him support by asking to meet him. He also tried to give support by talking to Brendan's girlfriend.

Brendan felt that someone cared about his situation. He trusted his friend and was willing to share his secrets with him.

The effect of educational experiences on growth and development

Education affects growth and development in a number of ways. Educational achievement affects job opportunities. The higher the level of educational achievement, the greater the range of jobs is available. Research has shown that people with a higher level of education tend to look after their health and the health of their children better.

Compulsory education in the United Kingdom is from 5–16 years of age. Many people stay on at school and college until they are 18 or 21 in order to get more qualifications and improve their job prospects.

Not only does education provide the opportunity to gain more knowledge and skills but it also widens our group of friends. We meet people at school and at college with whom we can share the same interests. Such friendships often become lifelong relationships. These support our emotional and social development.

The effect of employment and unemployment on growth and development

Having a job can have physical, intellectual, emotional and social benefits. A job provides an income. Some jobs involve some physical activity. Learning new tasks provides intellectual stimulation. What someone does for a living has an emotional aspect as it is an important part of their **self-concept**. There may be social contacts with workmates.

Someone who is unemployed does not have these things and looks for other ways of getting them. This could be through hobbies or voluntary work. Unemployment can affect a person by lowering their self-esteem and they may feel socially isolated.

> **Word check**
>
> **self-concept** – how we see or think about ourselves.

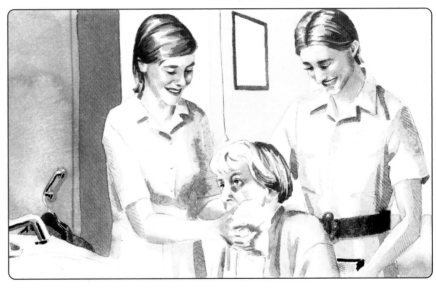

Learning new skills

The effect of ethnicity and religion on growth and development

Ethnicity and religion are part of someone's culture. Ethnicity is about the group that people feel they belong to, through nationality, religion, language and/or race. For instance, the inhabitants of a country may be of the same race and speak the same language, but if they follow different religions they may consider themselves as different ethnic groups.

If a number of people of the same ethnic group live in a country where the culture is different, they are called an ethnic minority group. Asian people from the Indian subcontinent think of themselves, for example, as Sikhs, Bangladeshis, Pakistanis or Indians. These are all different ethnic minority groups in the UK.

> **Word check**
>
> **ethnicity** – our cultural background.

Religion is often, but not always, part of ethnicity. It is a person's beliefs about the spiritual aspects of life. The main religion in the UK is Christianity, although only a minority of people go to church. Other major religions practised by ethnic minorities in this country are Islam, Sikhism, Hinduism, Buddhism, and Judaism.

When people are members of ethnic minority groups, their growth and development is often influenced by discrimination. This means being treated unfairly because of race, religion or some other factor.

20 What does ethnic minority mean?

Discrimination may affect people's life opportunities in a number of ways, even though there are laws to prevent this happening. Discrimination can affect many areas of our lives.

Access to education
People may have low expectations of people from some ethnic minority groups. As a result, they may not achieve as much in education as they could.

Access to employment
If employers discriminate against any group, people may find it more difficult to get a job. If they have a job, getting promotion may be a problem.

Access to health and social care services
Information about services may not be provided in a person's usual language. This can create barriers for them. Services may not be provided in a way that agrees with their custom or beliefs. They may have special dietary needs, for example, kosher food. They may have a cultural objection to being medically examined by a member of the opposite sex.

The effect of life experiences on growth and development

These are experiences such as birth, marriage, divorce and death. Between birth and death experiences affect our growth and development. Many people marry or have a long-term partner. They become responsible for one another and any children that they have.

A successful marriage or partnership promotes the development of both people through mutual support. On the other hand, some relationships are abusive. One partner may try to control the other, or use violence against them. These relationships can be very damaging to a person's development.

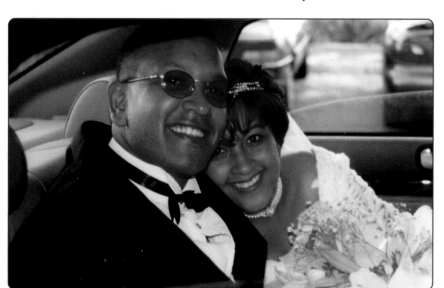

Just married

Ali

Ali is a Muslim who lives in England. He is the eldest child in a family of five. He is studying at sixth-form college to get qualifications so that he can train as a primary school teacher. His family are very supportive and have encouraged Ali as much as possible.

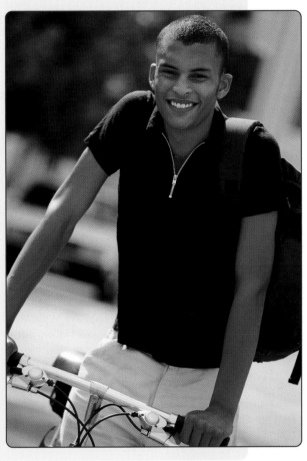

Ali has a small group of friends at the college with whom he gets on well. He does not go out with them at the weekend, because of his family and religious commitments. He would really like to go with them sometimes but he thinks that some of the people they meet might not accept him because of his culture.

Ali is very pleased when he passes his examinations and is accepted for teacher training. He then starts to worry about having to move away from home.

C1 What social and emotional factors are affecting Ali's growth and development?

C2 In what ways are Ali's friends not being sensitive to his cultural needs?

C3 Explain how Ali could help his friends to understand his cultural needs.

C4 How will Ali's educational experiences affect his growth and development?

Ali is 18

Key learning activity

K1 Describe THREE social factors that have influenced Ali's growth and development.

K2 Describe how Ali's family circumstances have influenced his emotional and social development.

K3 Explain how moving away to college is likely to affect Ali's emotional and social development.

Economic factors

When we talk about economic factors, we mean things to do with money. Health and well-being are affected by the amount of money we have. These are economic factors:

- income – which is usually from wages and private pensions, or state benefits such as child benefit, jobseeker's allowance, sickness and disability benefits, and the state retirement pension

- savings – when people have more money than they need to meet all their commitments they can save some

- essential bills – such as rent for housing, council taxes, gas, electricity and water bills, and transport costs

- debts – from borrowing money to buy a house (a mortgage) or an expensive piece of equipment, such as a washing machine, or from unpaid bills

- material possessions – the things that people buy to live comfortably, for example, a television or a car.

These are all important factors in human growth and development. The more money someone has, the more choices they have, and the better able they are to meet their physical needs.

Income

Someone with a high income can borrow money from a bank to buy a house, or can afford a high rent. They have a choice about the sort of house they live in and where it is. A person with a low income or no income at all may not be able to buy their own home. They may not have much choice about where they live. They may have to live in poor quality housing because they can only afford a low rent.

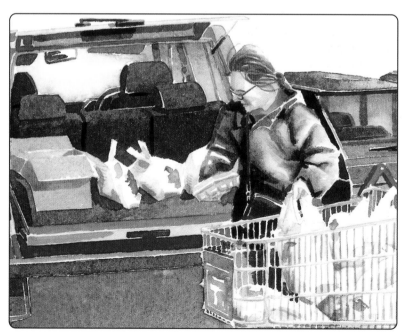

She can afford to buy what she wants for her family

Someone with a good income will probably have a car and be able to get to supermarkets where they can afford good quality food. People on low incomes often have to rely on public transport, which may not be convenient. They may have to buy food locally from small shops, and sometimes this will mean paying more.

People with a high income do not have to worry about fuel bills. They can meet their own physical needs and the needs of the people dependent on them. A person who has a low income may have to be more careful about the amount of gas and electricity that they use. They may not be able to keep their home as warm as they would like it. Keeping warm is important for families with young children, and for older people as they are more vulnerable to the cold.

Some people may not use their income wisely. They may put things like drink or cigarettes or drugs first before paying their bills. This could mean that eventually, because they owe so much money, they lose their homes and their family.

If a person on a high income is ill, and there is a waiting list for treatment under the National Health Service, then they may be able to afford private health care. Companies may provide private health care for their employees. People with lower incomes do not usually have the choice of private health care, they have to wait their turn on the waiting list.

Savings

Savings are important because they help people meet their needs. With some money in a bank or building society, they are prepared when something unexpected happens. If a vacuum cleaner breaks and has to be replaced, it is much easier for someone with savings. Without savings, people on a low income either have to go without or borrow money.

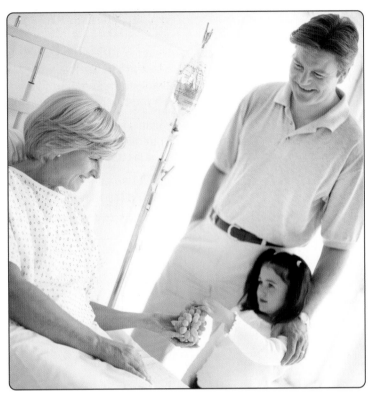

Private care: no waiting and good accommodation

Debts

Debts are important because they have to be paid. This means that less of our income is available to spend on things we need now.

Material possessions

Material possessions are important for meeting physical needs. Life is much more comfortable with appliances like cookers, vacuum cleaners and washing machines. Less essential things can add to the quality of people's lives, televisions and CD players, for example. Many people spend thousands of pounds on such things over the years. People on low incomes may not be able to do this.

Economic factors affect the way that people can meet their physical needs, but they also affect their intellectual, emotional and social needs. Being able to afford things can make us happy. Being unable to buy the things we need can make us unhappy and resentful. We may not want to invite people to our homes if we are ashamed of the condition of our furniture. This can mean that we have few friends and become socially isolated.

A parent on a low income might not be able to afford school trips that a parent on a high income can. People with higher incomes can also afford to help their children through higher education more easily. Parents' income can affect how well a child succeeds in education. Success in education improves a person's chances of getting a good job.

21 What is debt?

Our income and economic situation has an effect on all aspects of our growth and development.

Kevin

CASE STUDY

Kevin is 13. He lives with his family in rented council accommodation on an estate. Most of the families on the estate have low incomes. Kevin has three brothers between the ages of five and 11. His father works part-time in a shoe factory and his mother has a cleaning job at a school, which is also part-time.

Kevin's parents are very short of money. They have to pay the rent and they are in debt. They have to pay off some of what they owe for a car they once had. This leaves very little left for bills such as gas and electricity, or for food.

Kevin has asked if he can go on a school trip to the theatre one evening. It will cost £15 but his parents cannot afford for him to go. Kevin is really disappointed.

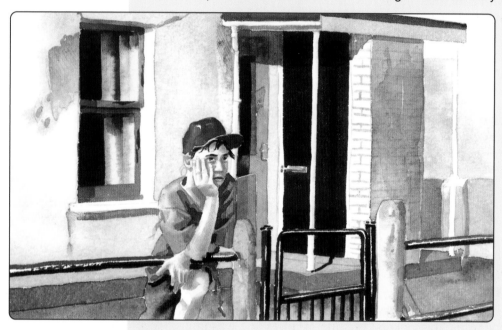

Kevin

C1 Give TWO economic factors that are affecting Kevin's growth and development.

C2 Identify THREE essential things that Kevin's family has to spend money on.

C3 How are the economic factors going to affect Kevin's growth and development?

Key learning activity

ACTIVITY

K1 Many of Kevin's classmates can afford designer clothes and have a computer at home. Kevin often does not have all the things he needs. How do you think this may affect Kevin's growth and development?

K2 Explain how poor housing and low income could affect Kevin's development.

K3 Explain how not being able to go on the school trip is going to affect Kevin's intellectual, emotional and social development.

Environmental factors

Environmental factors are the conditions people live in. They include:

- housing conditions
- pollution
- access to health and welfare services.

Housing conditions

We looked at some of the problems linked to housing in Unit 2. Turn back to page 148 to remind yourself of the information that was given.

Housing, see page 148 ➔

22 What is meant by inadequate housing?

Good quality housing usually has a positive effect on people and poor quality housing is more likely to have a negative effect. A high-rise flat may suit a single person, a couple without children, or older people who do not want a garden. It would not be very suitable for a single parent or couple with young children. Children need to be able to explore their surroundings to learn. If they cannot go outside to play, they do not get this opportunity.

Think about a poorly maintained high-rise flat in an area where there is a high crime rate and a lot of vandalism.

An infant being brought up there may suffer physical effects. If the flat is damp and difficult to heat, children are more likely to get respiratory illnesses that could affect their development.

There may be intellectual effects. If the flat is cramped, and it is not easy to get outside, the infant does not have a very stimulating environment to explore compared to an infant who lives in a house with a garden.

The infant's mother may suffer stress because of their poor living conditions and this may affect the way she handles the infant. This is likely to have emotional effects on the infant.

If the lift is often out of order the child will not have as many chances to meet other children and their social development may be affected.

Older people may also experience negative effects from living in a high-rise flat. If it is poorly maintained, damp and difficult to heat, they may be more at risk from respiratory illnesses or hypothermia. Older people often have less resistance to infection and have more difficulty maintaining their body temperature.

There may be emotional effects. If there is a high crime rate, such as burglaries or muggings, an older person may become anxious and suspicious of anybody who calls. Badly-maintained lifts may make it difficult for them to leave their flat. If the area looks frightening to them because there is graffiti or gangs of youths hanging around, then older people may be too scared to go out. This will have social effects. They will meet fewer people. They will not get the exercise they would if they were going out and walking, so it has physical effects, too.

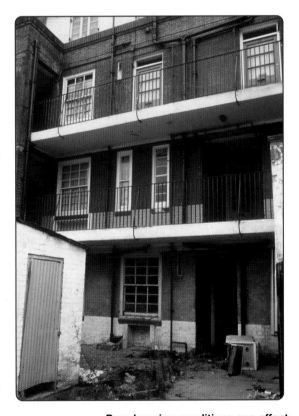

Poor housing conditions can affect our growth and development

The Robbins family

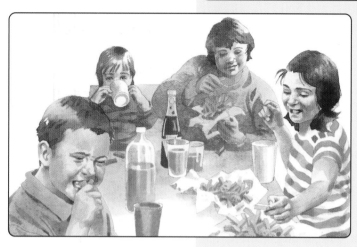

The Robbins family

Sue Robbins is a lone parent with three children, Jade aged one, Jody aged four and Connor aged six. They live in an upstairs flat in an old house with no access to the garden. The flat has been badly converted, has poor heating and the windows do not fit properly. The cooker is not working properly and the family often eat takeaway food.

The house is on a busy road, and the nearest park is a long way away. Sue is fed up and depressed. The children are boisterous and she is always yelling and shouting at them. Sometimes she hits them. Connor has missed a lot of school through illness. When he goes, his teacher often complains that he is unable to concentrate.

C1 Think about each member of the Robbins family. How are their physical, intellectual, emotional and social development being affected by their environment?

C2 Suggest ways in which the Robbins family could have support to help them in their present living conditions.

 Pollution, see page 149

Pollution

Pollution means the release of harmful things into the environment. Turn back to pages 149–152 to remind yourself about the information given there.

23 How can chemicals harm us?

Noise is often not thought of as a type of pollution, but it can be very harmful. Exposure to loud noise can cause deafness, and there are laws about how much noise a person can be exposed to in the workplace. Noise is produced by industry, transport and people going about their everyday lives. People who live near airports often complain about the noise of aircraft taking off. Busy roads and railway lines can be very noisy for people who live near them.

Noise can be caused by inconsiderate neighbours playing loud music or having late night parties. People may be particularly harmed by noise in their homes. It causes stress and may prevent them sleeping properly.

Access to health and welfare services

Access to health and welfare services is very important for people's health and well-being. If they have easy access, they are more likely to use preventative services, which will lower their chances of getting ill. If they do get ill they are more likely to get quick treatment and recover quickly.

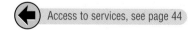 Access to services, see page 44

Turn back to pages 44–51 of Unit 1 to read about access to services and possible barriers.

24 What may prevent people from accessing health and social care services?

Effects of relationships on personal development

Getting started

During our lifetime we have many different types of relationships. In this section you will:

- find out about family relationships, including those with parents and siblings, and as parents of children
- find out about friendships and their effects on development
- understand the importance of intimate personal and sexual relationships
- find out about working relationships including teacher/student, employer/employee, peers and colleagues
- find out which relationships play a key part in an individual's social and emotional development at each life stage
- identify how these relationships can have a positive or negative effect on personal development
- identify the effect that abuse, neglect and lack of support can have on personal development.

These relationships could last a lifetime

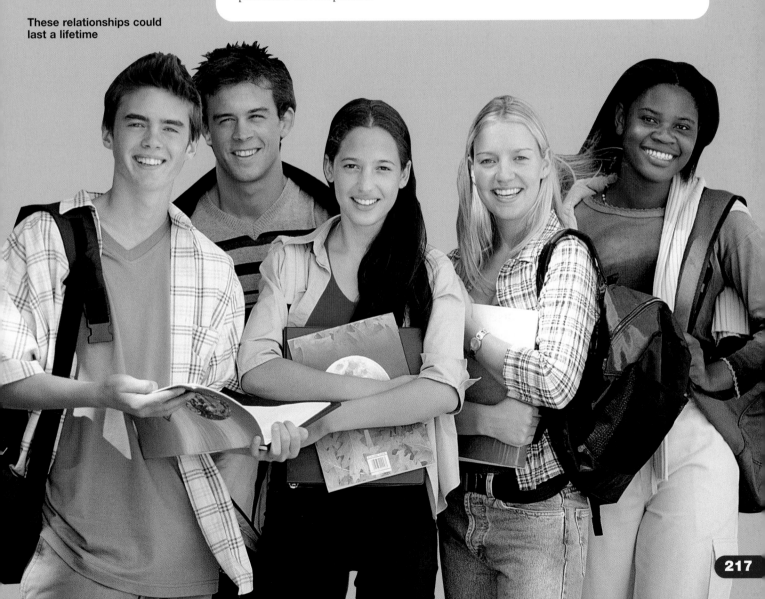

Family relationships

Most people will, at some time in their lives, live with or in a family. The family plays an important part in the development of individuals. How we feel about our family and how we get on with other family members influences the way we think and **relate** to people throughout our lives.

There are different types of family.

Nuclear famililes

A nuclear family of parents and children live as a self-contained family unit in a single household. When the children are young the whole family lives together. The parents share bringing up the children.

Lone parent families

A lone parent family is where one parent, either the mother or the father, is bringing up a child (or children) on their own. This could be because the parents have decided to separate or divorce, or one parent has died. Sometimes a mother decides that she wants to stay single and bring a child up on her own without support from the child's father. Sometimes a father leaves the mother and child.

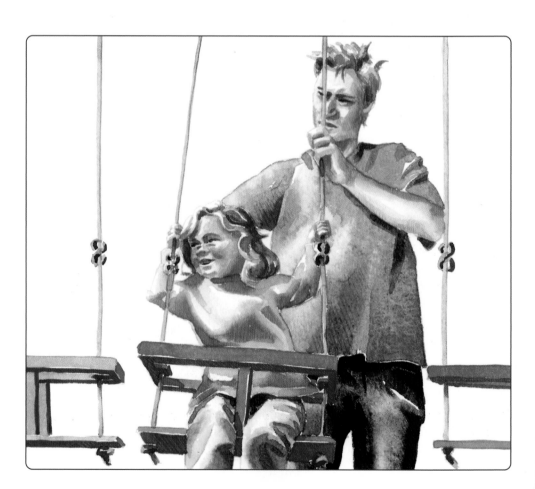

Being a single parent can be hard

Stepfamilies

A stepfamily results from remarriage after a divorce or the death of a parent. The child or children will be the natural child of one person in the marriage or partnership. An example of a stepfamily is:

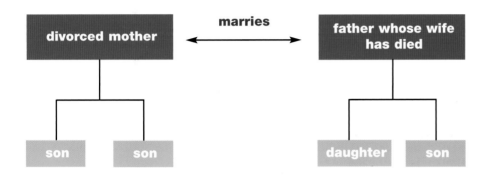

An example of a stepfamily

With increased early marriage breakdown many men and women separate and remarry new partners. They may have young children from previous marriages or relationships to care for. Children from different families in a stepfamily situation can find it hard to get on with one another in the early days of the new arrangement. This situation is usually resolved after the family settle down and become used to each other.

Extended families

An extended family is a large family group that includes parents, sisters, brothers, grandparents, uncles and aunts.

The members of the family all live together in the same building or close by. Such a large group can give support to each other by helping parents to bring up the children. They can give advice when there is a problem and help by contributing to the daily living expenses. Extended families are not now so common in western Europe as in other parts of the world.

Foster families

Foster families provide family life for children who cannot live with their natural parents. The foster parents try to make sure that the pattern of the children's life is as similar as possible to that of children who live with their own families.

Some children live in residential homes. These are usually adolescents who have serious problems and cannot be fostered. There may be six or seven children living with main carers.

25 Why do you think there are fewer extended families in western Europe now than there were in the past?

Word check

adoption – accepting responsibility for a child who is not one's own.

family ties – close links with family, loyalty.

Word check

provide – to give or make available.

biologically – how we function as human animals.

Word check

sexual partner – someone in an intimate physical relationship.

Word check

working relationship – the bond you make when you work with someone.

Families are made up of people of various ages who are usually related by birth or marriage. They can also be related through **adoption** into a family. Members of a family usually feel that they have special relationships with one another. These are often known as **family ties**.

26 What do you think makes family members feel they have something in common?

Each member of the family will have a number of different relationships. For example, as parents the mother and father **provide** for and support the family. They provide safe and secure surroundings for their children to grow up in. People can **biologically** become parents from the age of around 13, up to about 45–50 for women. However, most people are not ready to take on the care of another human being until they have a stable home and a strong relationship with their partner.

As **sexual partners** the mother and father develop intimate and loving relationships with each other.

One or both parents may go out to work. They will be an employee or an employer and have a **working relationship** with other people.

The parents can be friends with their children. They also have friends of their own age with whom they can talk and share activities.

27 Why do you think many people want to wait until they have a stable home before having a family?

Positive family relationships

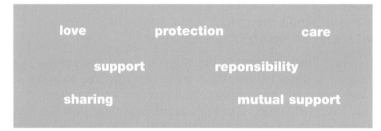

love   protection   care

support   reponsibility

sharing   mutual support

Text box

These are some features of a positive family relationship. Negative family relationships can develop for a variety of reasons, including:

- financial problems – lack of money can put a strain on relationships
- partners no longer in love and finding someone else to share their interests
- the death of a child – coping with such a bereavement can be very hard for parents
- children putting a strain on the parents' relationship.

When relationships break down, whether it is between adults or children or between children and adults, the people involved often get hurt.

The Patel family
CASE STUDY

Suresh Patel works as an environmental health officer and brings home a reasonable wage each month. Roopa works part time as a teacher. With their joint income, the family can afford to run a car and they are buying their semi-detached house. They also have enough money for outings for the children and holidays. The Patels have bought an outdoor slide, a swing and trampoline for the children to play on. They have made sure that each play item is put up properly and is securely fixed to the ground. After the family have had their evening meal Suresh and Roopa always spend time playing with the children. The children tell their parents what they have done during the day and they tell the children something about the things they have been doing. Before they go to bed the children have a story read to them and their mum and dad give them both a big hug.

Features of relationships
ACTIVITY

A1 Look up the meaning of each word given in the text box on page 220. Write down the word and its meaning.

A2 From the case study select an example to show how Suresh and Roopa showed the following features in their relationship with their children:

- protection
- love
- friendship
- providing.
- sharing

A3 Write a short case study of your own based on a family with a teenage son. You should make sure that you have included examples of how the family:

- provide support
- share.
- give protection

A4 Exchange case studies with another person in the group. For the case study you have now, write down examples of providing support, protection and sharing.

Key learning activity

K1 Write down TWO features of Suresh and Roopa's relationship:

- jealousy
- hatred
- physical attraction
- support.

K2 Describe how Suresh and Roopa are showing mutual support in their relationship.

K3 Explain how a loving and caring relationship is likely to affect the development of the two children.

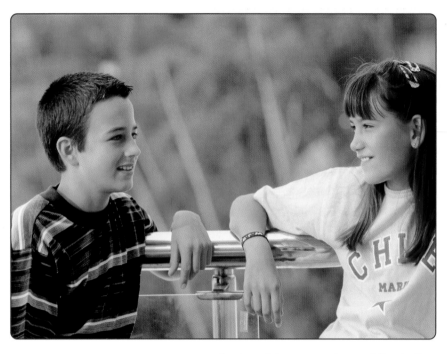

Brothers and sisters are siblings

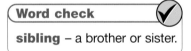

Word check ✓

sibling – a brother or sister.

Siblings

Sibling is another way of saying brother or sister. They are children who are in the same family. Most people who have siblings are very protective towards them. They may quarrel from time to time but they would not want any harm to come to their siblings.

When a new baby is born into the family an older sibling, who may previously have been the only child, can become jealous. Jealousy can be shown in many ways, such as snatching a toy away from the new baby, behaving badly, having a temper tantrum or demanding attention. It is in these situations that parents need to remember to give love and support to the child who is jealous.

Relationships experienced by infants

When they are first born babies start to develop very close relationships with their mother and then their father. This is known as 'bonding'. As a child grows and develops it will form relationships with a much wider group of people.

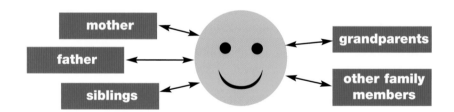

An infant's relationships

By the time the child reaches the age of eight years the relationships it has with others will have widened quite a lot. For example:

- mother and father
- siblings
- grandparents
- other family members, such as aunts and uncles
- playgroup leaders
- other children
- teachers
- neighbours
- parents of their friends.

Sheema ⬤ CASE STUDY

Sheema is eight years old. She plays with her four year-old brother while her mother gets their breakfast. She can dress herself and get ready to go to school. On some mornings she quarrels with her mother because she wants to take dolls and toys to school with her. She wants to take far too many.

Sheema's mother walks with her to school each day. As soon as they reach the school gate she runs off to meet her friends. She enjoys school and likes the work she has to do. Her teacher is pleased with what she does. Sheema cooperates well with her teacher and tries hard with her work.

After school, Sheema, her mum and brother call at the local shop. Sheema has pocket money to spend and likes to choose her own sweets. Sometimes she shares them with her brother.

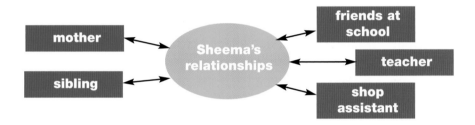

Some of the features of these relationships show that Sheema:

- has become less dependent on her parents
- has become more independent
- is more confident
- is more cooperative
- is more sociable.

Features of Sheema's relationships ⬤ ACTIVITY

A1 From the case study identify examples to show the following features:

- independence
- confidence
- being more sociable
- being less dependent.

A2 Explain how Sheema's mother still provides protection for her daughter.

A3 Describe the relationship between Sheema and her teacher.

A4 How is going to school likely to affect Sheema's development?

Key learning activity

ACTIVITY

K1 From the four factors given below, write down TWO features of the relationship between Sheema and her teacher:

- power
- cooperation
- sexual
- jealousy.

K2 Describe THREE ways that Sheema's relationship with her friends could affect her development.

K3 Think about Sheema's personal development. How could her mother help her to become more independent but still protect her from harm.

Friendships

Friendships support our need to have **companionship** and boost our self-esteem. There can be different types of friendships such as:

- close friends – people you trust and share secrets with; you are likely to share the same interests and do things together

- other friends – people you like that you might meet quite often but you will probably not share things with them that are confidential or secret

- associates – people you meet from time to time, perhaps at school or college, at work, perhaps in your social activities

- acquaintances – people you say hello to when you see them, but would not spend long periods of time with.

28 What do you think are the qualities of a close friend?

Making friends

Friendships are often formed when we are physically attracted to a person and when we like the way they do things. We may like their personality, for example, their sense of humour, the fact that they are **dependable** or the way they are prepared to work together on school work or hobbies.

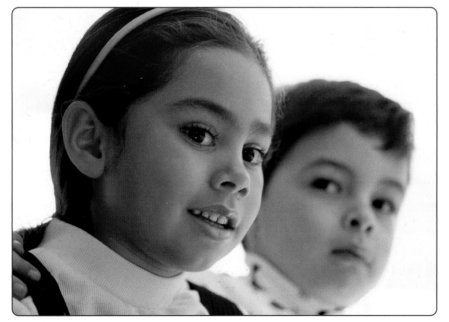

Friendships can start quite early

In friendships people **communicate** with one another. Communication skills enable us to express our feelings and emotions to each other and to share information. Some people define friendship as 'groups of people who come together voluntarily'. Features of friendships are:

- sharing
- being honest with one another
- trusting each other
- providing mutual support
- giving **reassurance**
- providing stimulation
- making each other feel valued as individuals
- loyalty.

Teenage girls can develop very deep and **intense** friendships with other girls. These relationships do not always last as jealousy and **disloyalty** may get in the way. Teenage boys often seek the company of other boys who have the same interests. They sometimes like being in a large group of friends, while girls of a similar age prefer to be in smaller groups.

Both boys and girls are influenced quite strongly by their peers at this stage of their development. This is known as peer pressure. Some teenagers will not, for example, answer a question in class if they think it would make them look too enthusiastic to their peers.

Word check
communicate – transfer information between two individuals.

Word check
reassurance – convincing a person effectively.

Word check
intense – strong. **disloyalty** – something that could cause you not to be trusted.

29 Why do you think boys like to be in larger groups and girls prefer to be with small groups of friends?

Adolescents often have disagreements with their parents and appear to 'break' friends with the family. This is usually because they want to be more independent and make their own decisions. Most quarrels with parents are only temporary and soon made up. However, some disagreements may lead to the adolescent leaving home because the relationship between the teenager and parents has broken down.

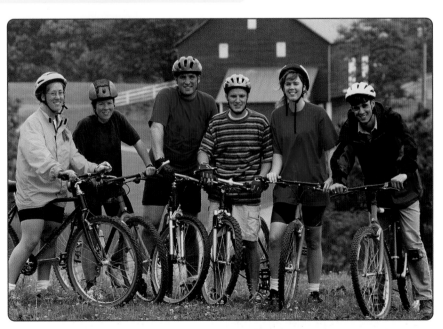

Sharing the same interests

Adult friendships

Adult friendships can be more lasting than when we are young. For example, we could become friends with our immediate neighbours. This might just be by speaking when we see each other. Sometimes neighbours can develop close friendships and do a lot together.

People with whom we work can also become friends. We may enjoy going out with a group of people from work to a concert or for a shopping trip or to a football match.

When people retire from work they often miss the company and the friendships of their work colleagues. They may decide to have a pet to keep them company. By having a dog, for example, older adults may make new friends as they are likely to take the dog out for walks. While walking the dog they may stop to speak to people. They may take their dog to training classes and make new friends through such activities.

30 How are adolescent friendships different from those formed by adults?

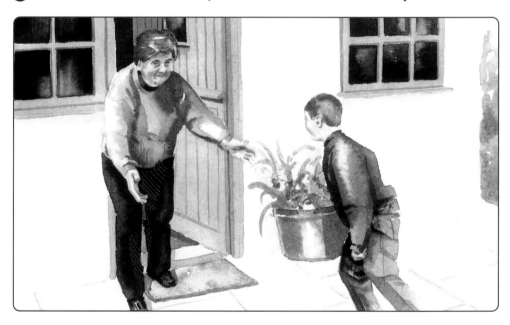

Going to stay with Granny

Older adults often form friendships with their grandchildren. They may help to look after them while the parents are at work or in the evening, if they live close enough. Some have their grandchildren to stay for holidays and firm friendships are formed that last as the children grow into adults.

As time passes, older adults lose some of their friends through illness or death. This can make them feel lonely and isolated. As they themselves get older, they may not be able to travel as much as they used to do to meet their friends. They may also have to cope with the death of a lifelong partner who was a very close friend.

31 What do you think might be the effect of losing a lifelong partner who has been a friend?

Zac

Zac is 72. He used to live with his two brothers but they have both died and now he is on his own. When his brothers were alive Zac did the cooking and kept the house tidy. The brothers could not help because they were ill. Zac used to read the newspaper to them. In the evening they would play chess or dominoes.

Zac now has mobility problems and cannot walk very far. He used to visit his friend Rob every day. Rob lives two streets away. Rob cannot visit Zac either as he has Parkinson's disease and cannot go out. When they were able to meet they used to spend a long time chatting and would enjoy a game of cards and a pint together.

A home care assistant visits Zac twice each week to help keep the house tidy. A social worker has arranged for a volunteer to visit Zac to chat to him on three evenings each week.

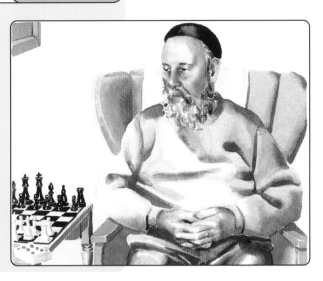

Zac is unable to get out to meet his friends

Changes in relationships ACTIVITY

A1 Think about the relationship changes that Zac has had in this life stage. Give THREE examples of the changes that have occurred. For each change explain the effect you think they would have on Zac.

A2 Zac used to enjoy meeting his friend Rob. Copy and complete the chart to show how each feature was shown in their relationship.

Feature of the relationship	How it was shown between Zac and Rob
Sharing	
Mutual support	
Loyalty	
Dependency	

A3 A volunteer friend plans to visit Zac each week. Describe THREE features that could develop in this relationship.

A4 Explain the effect on Zac's relationships of not been able to go out so often.

A5 What other actions could be taken by the social worker to widen Zac's relationships? How would they help?

Key learning activity

K1 Describe TWO features of Zac's relationship with the home care assistant.

K2 Describe the features of Zac's relationship with his brothers when they were alive.

K3 Explain how having a wider circle of friends could help Zac.

Intimate personal and sexual relationships

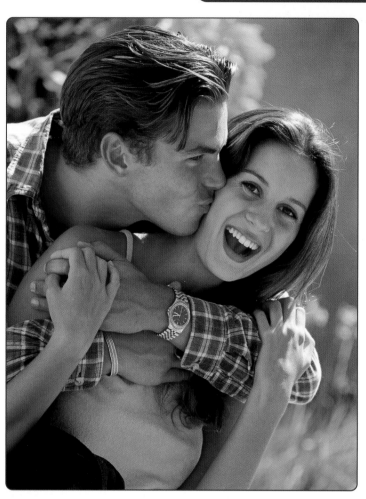

Very much in love

There are many different kinds of love. We use the word 'love' quite often. For example, we might say 'I love my dog' or 'I love going on holiday' or 'I love my dad'. The love we feel for a girlfriend or boyfriend is a different type of love than the love we have for our family and friends. This is because there is sexual attraction.

Intimate relationships involve being very close to someone. Our sexual feelings start to develop during the early teens. This means that teenagers can fall in and out of love quite often. These early relationships often do not last because adolescents may not have matured sufficiently to be sensitive to the needs of others. Falling in and out of love, however, can be a very painful experience!

Sexual love often begins with physical attraction. Two people may find, as they get to know one another better, that they have the same interests. The relationship may deepen and sexual love develops out of a close friendship. Sexual activity is one of the most powerful expressions of intimacy that two people can share.

> **Word check**
>
> **intimate relationship** – a very close and trusting relationship.

> **Word check**
>
> **role model** – someone we observe or copy.

Learning to form sexual relationships

Our parents are often **role models** on which we base our own relationships. Touch plays an important role in sexual activity. Warm and friendly touches that show care and concern for one another are different from the very physical kissing and cuddling that happen in sexual relationships. Touch is the main language of sexual relationships when falling in love. Sexual intercourse is the expression of emotional and physical attraction.

Adults learn to be sensitive to the needs of others. As a result they are less likely to be thinking about themselves but, instead consider the best interests of the other person. Both people in the relationship are considering the needs of the other person first. As a result the relationship is more likely to last.

32 Why is it necessary to be sensitive to the needs of a partner?

Working relationships

We spend quite a lot of our adult life working. The relationships that we form with people while we are working are an important part of our lives. Working relationships are different from other relationships, such as friendships, because they have a specific purpose. In some working relationships one person is in a position of power over another.

Working relationships can include, for example:

- student and teacher
- peers
- employer and employee
- colleagues.

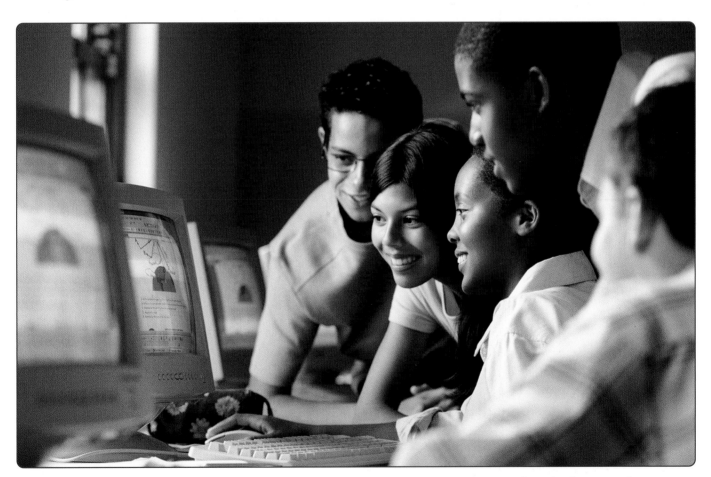

Learning to cooperate

Student/teacher relationships

As early as five years of age, or even before if a child attends a day nursery, children learn to work with other people, both adults and other children. Learning to work with others means learning to **cooperate**. A nursery nurse or teacher may ask a child to do something. The child does what has been asked and a working relationship has been formed.

> **Word check**
>
> **cooperate** – to work together.

Another feature of a working relationship is trust. This is particularly true when working relationships are made with children, for example, as a teacher. The child is dependent on the teacher and trusts the adult not to harm them in any way.

Adolescents studying for examinations are also working with teachers and lecturers. A feature of this type of relationship is a **partnership**. The student and the teacher work closely together exchanging knowledge and ideas. There is power in the relationship as the teacher or lecturer is in charge. A student may also want advice on a problem from a form teacher or personal tutor. They would share confidential information.

Peer relationships

Students also have working relationships with their peers. They may work on a project with one or more people in their class. In this situation none of the people is in charge, although sometimes one person will take a **leadership role**. Peers can have a very strong effect on the actions we take. This is known as peer pressure.

Peers are usually around the same age as ourselves and can influence us in good ways or in bad ways. This is known as having a positive or negative influence. Working relationships with teachers and lecturers can be greatly influenced by the attitudes of our peers.

33 Why do you think peers influence our behaviour?

Employer/employee relationships and colleagues

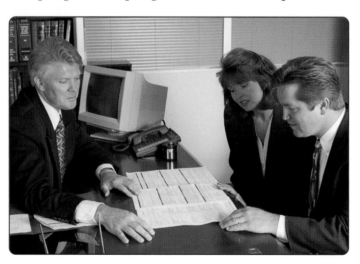

Following the employer's instruction is important

Not many people are able to choose the people they work with.

Good working relationships help to keep employees and employers happy and this contributes to good health. Good communication is a feature of successful working relationships. Friendships can develop between colleagues who are working on the same tasks or who have the same job status.

> **Word check** ✓
>
> **partnership** – relationship involving two or more individuals.

> **Word check** ✓
>
> **leadership role** – activity carried out by someone who leads or is in charge.

It is more unusual for people who work at different levels or who have a different status within an organisation to make deep friendships with each other. This is because there is often an 'invisible barrier' between staff levels. For example, a manager or supervisor who is friendly with a care assistant could not easily reprimand the care assistant if this became necessary. It is not often that a person in charge of a department shares a problem they may have with a junior member of staff. This is because they may feel that the junior will think they are not able to cope.

A good atmosphere in the workplace depends on **mutual tolerance** and valuing the contribution that others are making. An employee who shows respect for another employee is likely to be respected in return. An employee who shows respect for the employer is likely to receive back that respect.

Some employees may feel that an employer has power over them. They may desperately need the work because they have a mortgage and bills to pay. They may feel that they have to do whatever their employer asks in order to keep their job. This type of attitude does not help to make good working relationships.

> **Word check**
>
> **mutual tolerance** – where two or more people accept what the other is doing and have respect for their opinions.

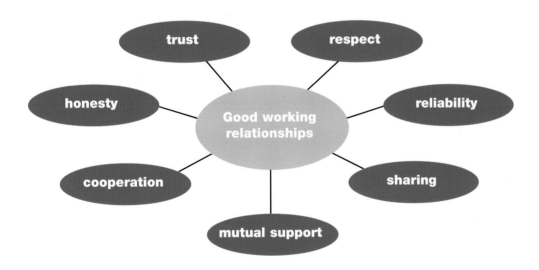

If these are present in a good working relationship the effects will be:

- higher self-esteem
- positive self-image
- shared skills
- sense of self-worth
- strong sense of identity.

Hebbi CASE STUDY

Hebbi has been a nurse at the same hospital for 20 years. She used to enjoy her work, but now she finds it quite hard as so much is expected of her. She never seems to have enough staff, equipment or materials. She has made many requests for more resources, but her line manager has been unable to provide them.

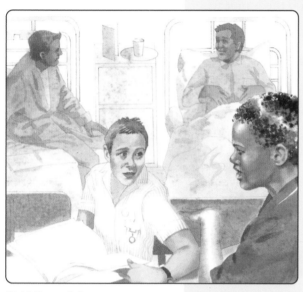

When she first started at the hospital Hebbi was happy. She liked the people she worked with, as they were able to talk about things together. Sometimes they went out as a group in the evenings. They always has a good time and seemed to laugh a lot. At work they all helped one another, particularly if someone needed help to manage their workload.

Now she is a sister she feels that she cannot be quite so friendly with the other nurses. She expects them to do a good job and will not allow standards on her ward to fall. There are one or two staff that she would, if she could choose, prefer not to work with. She knows, however, that in her professional role she needs to treat her staff equally.

Hebbi's work is important to her. She is divorced and has a mortgage to pay. Her children are at university and they are always needing more books or help in paying for their accommodation.

Hebbi's work is important to her

Hebbi ACTIVITY

A1 From the case study show how Hebbi demonstrates the following features in her relationships:

- mutual support
- loyalty
- sharing
- respect.
- dependency

A2 Explain how Hebbi shows that she values those with whom she works.

A3 What effect could financial pressures have on Hebbi's relationships at work and with her family?

A4 If Hebbi gave up work how might her relationships with her children change?

- How do you think this would affect Hebbi?

Key learning activity

K1 What was an unexpected life event that Hebbi experienced?

K2 Hebbi works as a sister in a hospital ward. Describe the main features of her relationship with her present staff.

K3 Hebbi was happy during her early working life. How do you think this affected her personal development?

The effects of positive and negative relationships

During our lives we experience both positive and negative relationships and these affect us in different ways.

Positive relationships help us to have a good self-image. A negative relationship is likely to lower our self-esteem, make us have doubts and lessen our confidence.

Positive relationships

A positive relationship can mean:

- having someone to share an interest
- knowing that you are loved and liked
- having someone for whom you can provide support in times of stress
- having someone to support you when you need help.

Positive relationships are essential if we are to have a high self-esteem. We need to feel good about ourselves. This happens when we feel we are valued. For example, we feel valued when someone tells us we have done a job well. We feel good in ourselves because we know we have achieved the task that has been set and this gives us a good feeling of self-worth.

Good relationships contribute to our own sense of identity and help us to know about the direction in which we are going.

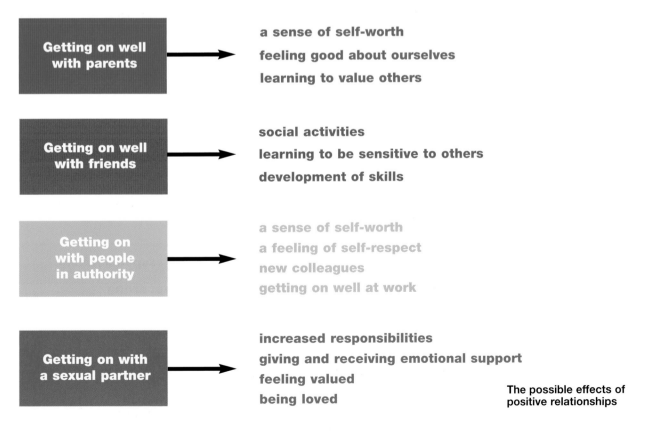

| Getting on well with parents | → | a sense of self-worth
feeling good about ourselves
learning to value others |

| Getting on well with friends | → | social activities
learning to be sensitive to others
development of skills |

| Getting on with people in authority | → | a sense of self-worth
a feeling of self-respect
new colleagues
getting on well at work |

| Getting on with a sexual partner | → | increased responsibilities
giving and receiving emotional support
feeling valued
being loved |

The possible effects of positive relationships

Negative relationships

Negative or poor relationships are likely, after a period of time, to contribute to poor health. Negative relationships mean being unable to get on with other people. We may find it difficult to get on with our family or our friends, or with people in authority. It may be that we find it difficult to get on with any other people. When we do not get on with others we are likely to become socially isolated. We resist joining in activities or meeting other people. Our sense of identity and self-esteem is affected. We may find that we fail in the tasks that we are given to do. This could lead to poor examination results or loss of a job. We may not be able to pay our bills or eat properly. This could even result in becoming homeless, poor health and turning to crime in order to get money.

None of these examples will help us to be successful in our lives.

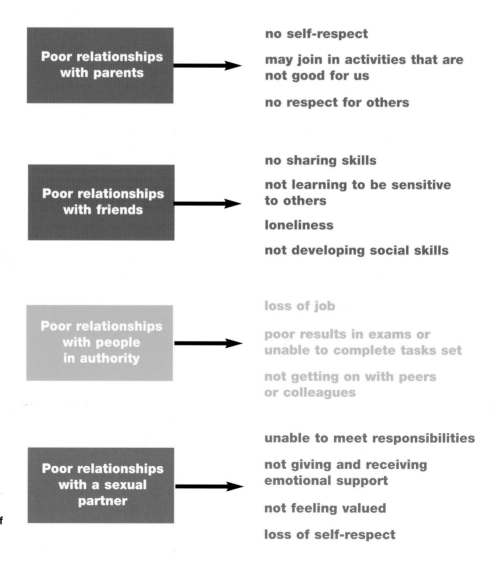

The possible effects of negative relationships

Poor relationships with parents →
- no self-respect
- may join in activities that are not good for us
- no respect for others

Poor relationships with friends →
- no sharing skills
- not learning to be sensitive to others
- loneliness
- not developing social skills

Poor relationships with people in authority →
- loss of job
- poor results in exams or unable to complete tasks set
- not getting on with peers or colleagues

Poor relationships with a sexual partner →
- unable to meet responsibilities
- not giving and receiving emotional support
- not feeling valued
- loss of self-respect

The effect of abuse, neglect and personal support

Abuse can take various forms, including:

- physical abuse – being hit

- sexual abuse – being raped or assaulted

- verbal abuse – being shouted at or insulted

- emotional abuse – being made to feel that we have no value, constantly criticised or belittled.

Being abused in any way at all will probably lead to very negative feelings and a poor opinion of ourselves. It is likely that we will not be able to form good relationships with others. We may be affected by becoming withdrawn, quiet, unsociable, angry and resentful. It is likely that we will not cooperate with others. We may start bullying other people who are weaker than ourselves. The effects of such behaviour will make us become disliked by our friends and people will want to avoid us.

Without the support of parents, friends, teachers, employers, partners we are unlikely to be able to form positive relationships.

Darren
CASE STUDY

Darren is 15. He is always quarrelling with his family. He never seems able to please them. His examination results are never good enough. His parents do not like his friends. They do not approve of the clothes he chooses.

To stop the arguments Darren stays out late at night. He is then tired the next day and falls asleep during lessons. He is not managing to keep up with his work. His teacher keeps him behind for detention to catch up.

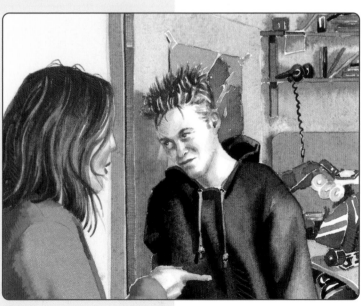

Darren begins to hang around more with his one friend. He does not really feel happy. His friend persuades him to help him break into a car. Darren knows this is wrong but he does it to please his friend.

The next day the police call at Darren's home. Darren has been traced as being one of the people who has broken into the car.

When Darren and his parents return from the police station the most awful row starts. Darren packs a bag and leaves home.

Darren is 15

Darren ACTIVITY

A1 Darren's relationship with his parents is poor. Describe the effect that this is likely to have on his personal development.

A2 How is Darren's friend affecting his personal development?

A3 Explain how Darren's parents could have provided support to prevent relationships becoming so poor.

A4 How do you think Darren felt after he left home?

Key learning activity

K1 Write down TWO features of a positive relationship:

- arguing
- jealousy
- sharing
- being valued.

K2 Describe the features of a positive relationship.

K3 Explain how Darren's relationship with his teacher could affect his self-esteem.

K4 How do you think Darren's future development is likely to be affected by the negative relationships he experienced at 15?

Self-concept

Getting started

We all have a picture of ourselves – who we are, what we are like inside. This is the image of ourselves that we like others to see. This is called our self-concept. It is based on two things:

- what we believe we are like as a person
- what we believe that other people think about us.

In this section we will find out about how a person's self-concept is affected by factors such as their:

- age
- appearance
- gender
- culture
- emotional development

- education
- relationships with others
- sexual orientation
- life experiences.

Projecting a positive self-image

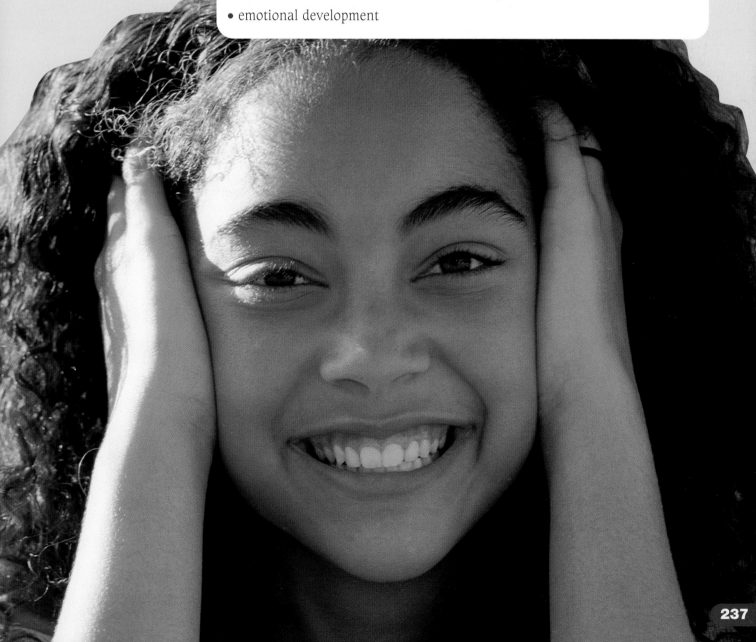

What is self-concept?

Word check ✓

self-awareness – knowing ourselves, including our strengths and weaknesses.

Self-concept means understanding ourselves. To understand ourselves we must first of all have developed **self-awareness**, but how do we do this?

To develop self-awareness we need to build up a picture of ourselves, using:

- the knowledge we have about ourselves
- the feedback we receive from other people.

Self-concept is part of our emotional and social development. The view we have of ourselves changes as a result of the experiences we have, life events, and the life stage we are in. Self-concept is like a 'self-portrait', the image that we have of ourselves. Having a clear picture about who we are and how we feel about ourselves helps us to feel happy, safe and secure. This good feeling about ourselves gives us a high self-esteem. High self-esteem helps us to relate more easily to the people we meet, such as our family, friends and others. This gives us a positive self-concept. A person with a good self-concept will generally view life experiences positively. They value themselves as a person. If we think we are valuable, we will expect other people to value us.

If we have a poor self-concept, we are not going to feel good about ourselves and have low self-esteem. This poor picture of ourselves can mean that we may not get on well with others. We may feel that others do not value us. This may make us feel that we are unable to make a worthwhile contribution to society. The result is a very low opinion of ourselves and a poor self-portrait.

34 Think about yourself. Have you a high or low self-concept? Give reasons for your answer.

Knowing how we feel about ourselves is an emotional factor. If we feel proud about our skills and the achievements we have made, such as being good at a particular sport, or a particular subject, we are likely to have a high self-esteem. If we are ashamed of our behaviour or we do not like the way we look, we are likely to have negative feelings about ourselves. We will probably develop a low self-esteem.

35 Have you any points that you do not like about yourself?

Age

Our self-concept changes according to our age and the life stage we are in. An important part of our self-concept is what we believe other people think about us. We learn this from infancy, and it is an important part of our emotional development. If we have been treated harshly, or abused as a young child, we may grow up with a poor sense of our own worth.

George Mead, a theorist, thought that children's behaviour developed because of their ability to imitate adult behaviour and because they had the ability to imagine characters. A child of two might in their play pretend to be a cat or a dog. They do not need to understand what cats and dogs are, they just copy the actions and the sounds they have seen them make.

In later development, around four years, a child might begin to imitate adult behaviour. For example, Isobel, aged four was given some dolls and a pushchair for her birthday. She dressed the dolls in coats and put on their shoes, gloves and hats. She put them in the pushchair and strapped them in. Then she put on her own coat and pretended to leave the house with a shopping bag and the pushchair with the dolls.

Isobel was just copying what she had seen her parents do. She was imagining a character or person. Mead believed that this was the beginning of the character of 'me' – Isobel's own self-image.

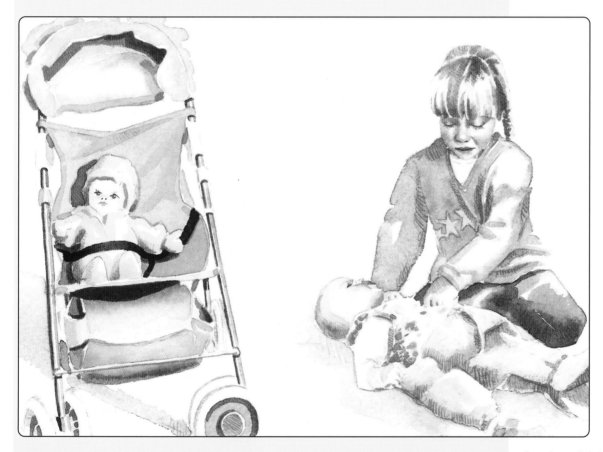

Copying adult behaviour

36 How does Mead think children start to develop self-awareness?

Self-concept in infancy and childhood

A newborn baby has no concept of itself as a person. Babies need to develop emotionally before they can understand that other people have feelings of their own. Until they understand this, they cannot understand that other individuals have opinions about them. This is why young children cannot play cooperatively with others, and why the infant having a tantrum in the street is not embarrassed to lie on the floor kicking and screaming.

A very young baby is helpless and depends on carers to meet all their needs. Whether they are treated kindly, neglectfully or harshly affects how they think about the world and how it values them.

As children get older, they meet a wider range of people. These people start to influence the picture they are forming of themselves, their self-portrait. They are strongly influenced by their family and the friends they make. They learn that they have to fit in with others. They learn basic social rules and values.

When a child does something well they are usually praised. When they do something that is unacceptable, they are usually told off. In this way the child adds to the picture they are developing of themselves.

Children do not just do the things they are taught or imitate what they see happening around them. They think about what is happening and decide what their own values are. This is called internalising or examining within themselves the experiences they are having.

37 How does a child add to the picture they have of themselves?

Self-concept in adolescence

An adolescent's sense of self is very strong. Adolescents want more independence. They want to make their own decisions. They may not feel very secure in making these decisions but they have an internal picture of themselves that they try to project so that others can see who they are. Adolescents often identify themselves by their membership of particular groups.

A good self-awareness helps adolescents develop a secure sense of self. They need this in order to:

• make difficult decisions

• form social and sexual relationships

• develop confidence in work roles or in a chosen college course.

The illustration on the next page shows some of the people who might influence the development of an adolescent's self-concept.

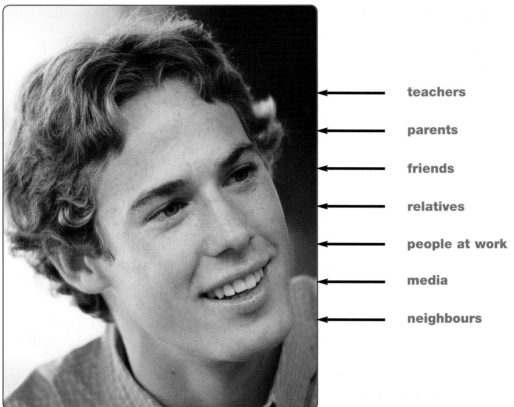

teachers

parents

friends

relatives

people at work

media

neighbours

**Teenagers are affected
by many influences**

38 What else might influence the development of self-concept?

Self-concept in adulthood

How we learn to value ourselves in childhood and during adolescence can affect us as adults. Adults are recognised by society as being fully independent and responsible for all their actions. We are surrounded by images of young, attractive people in advertisements, newspapers and other media. These can greatly influence our internal image of how we think we should be.

In older adulthood it is important that we still keep a clear sense of our self-concept. The image that we have of ourselves is influenced by the life events we have experienced. Events that influence self-concept might include marriage, starting a family or experiencing divorce, for example. Some of these life events reinforce the positive image we may have of ourselves. Others may have a negative effect. A few people may experience accidents that change their lives. From being able-bodied they may become disabled. This can be very challenging and sometimes it can be very hard to keep a positive self-image in these circumstances.

39 Why might it be hard to keep a positive self-image if you were disabled as a result of an accident?

Leroy

Leroy, 37, is a college lecturer. He has a wife and three children, aged eight, five and three. Leroy's wife works part time as a teacher. The family are always very busy. They take the children to and from school and to their various clubs and activities during the evenings and weekends. They are a happy family.

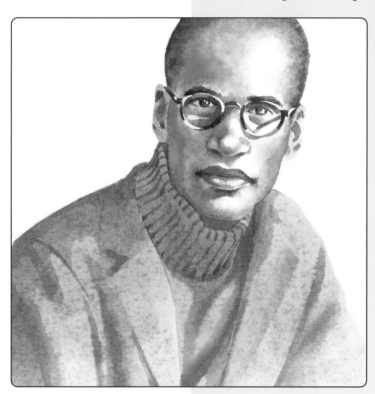

Leroy was a happy, healthy man before his accident

Leroy cycles to college to make sure he gets enough exercise. On the way home one day he is knocked off his bicycle by a car. He is taken to hospital with spinal injuries. He has a three-hour operation to remove pieces of bone from his spinal cord.

Three months after the accident Leroy is told that he will never be able to work again. He can shuffle around the downstairs rooms at home but he cannot walk properly. He cannot get upstairs and he is in pain most of the time. He cannot work at his computer for longer than 10 minutes because of the pain. The worst thing for him is being unable to help his wife with the daily jobs or play with the children.

Leroy becomes very depressed about his state of health.

Leroy

A1 How has Leroy's intellectual development been affected by the accident?

A2 How do you think Leroy's self-concept is affected as a result of the accident?

A3 How do you think the accident will affect Leroy's wife's self-concept?

Key learning activity

K1 Explain how the self-concept of Leroy's children could be affected as a result of the accident.

K2 Assess the possible effects Leroy's accident could have on his self-concept in the future.

Middle age

From the age of 50 people may experience discrimination in the workplace. Some employers prefer younger staff that they may see as being more flexible and adaptable. People over 50 may feel that they are not valued as much as younger people. A person with a strong self-concept would probably find other areas of their lives where they are valued, such as being a member of a club or the leader of a committee. They could still be affected in some way by the discrimination, however. They may:

- feel hurt

- feel they are not valued

- feel rejected

- become resentful and angry.

If someone's self-concept has been lowered the effect may be that they withdraw from social activities for fear of getting hurt again. They may not want to trust people. They may communicate less with others. In some circumstances they may become so angry that they physically hurt the person closest to them.

Such actions contribute to developing a negative self-concept. They may need help to see themselves in a different way and to cope with the situation.

Older adults

In late adulthood some people feel that they are not valued, particularly as they have lost their work role. They may become withdrawn and depressed. They may feel that others think they have nothing to contribute.

Ian   CASE STUDY

Ian is 63. He has worked as a salesman in a furniture store for 30 years. Ian loves his work. He lives on his own so he enjoys meeting the customers and chatting to his colleagues. Sometimes he goes out with his work colleagues for a drink and a game of darts. This is his main social life.

He is called in to see the manager when he arrives at work one day. The manager tells Ian that the firm would like him to take early retirement. This is because they are going to introduce a number of changes and feel that Ian would benefit financially if he were to leave at the end of the month.

The manager makes it clear that he expects Ian to accept the package being offered.

C1 How will Ian's social development be affected by taking early retirement?

C2 How do you think Ian's self-concept might be affected by taking early retirement?

Appearance

Appearance means what we look like, and it is very important to us.

Faces are a significant part of our appearance. We use them to recognise, and communicate with, other people. The very first thing that a baby recognises is the shape of a face. Once we start talking, our facial expressions are a major means of communication. They tell other people what we are feeling, and often show a more honest picture of our inner thoughts than the words we speak.

So, if something happens to a person's face, it can have serious emotional effects. Someone's face could be changed by being badly burned, or by an operation. A stroke stops them making facial expressions. People who have experienced this often say that they do not feel like the same person. For similar reasons, any congenital defect that affects someone's face, such as a birthmark, can have serious emotional effects. Acne is a common problem for adolescents, which often makes them very self-conscious.

One way we judge a person's age is from their face. Many people are quite happy with their appearance as they age. Sometimes a person's age has a negative effect on their self-concept. They may want to try to remove the signs of ageing. There are a large number of expensive cosmetics that claim to do this. Some people have cosmetic surgery to try to stop the signs of ageing.

40 How does the appearance of a person's face influence their self-concept?

> **Word check**
>
> **gender role** – how men and women are expected to act in particular situations.

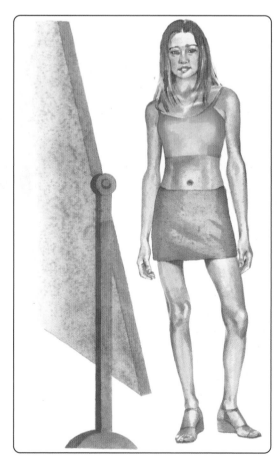

"I wish I could be thinner."

Body shape

Body shape can be very important to self-concept. Adolescent girls particularly may think that they have to be thin to be attractive. Some adolescents think of themselves as fat and unattractive because they do not meet these ideals.

In some cases, their image of themselves becomes so distorted that they develop eating disorders such as anorexia nervosa. People with this disorder become unhealthily thin but cannot see this because they have a distorted image of their body. Some boys have similar anxieties about their bodies and exercise to change their body shape.

41 How can clothes influence our self-concept?

Gender

Gender is not the same as sex. Someone's sex is determined by their genes. Gender is about the way society expects individuals of each sex to behave. Gender affects self-concept because individuals have to learn how other people expect someone of their sex to behave. This is called a **gender role**. There are two ways that children learn what is expected of individuals of their gender.

Social learning theory

Children watch and copy the people around them. This is called role modelling. This explanation of how we learn how to behave is called **social learning theory**.

Behaviourist theory

Children see how people react to their behaviour. They learn that some actions win approval and some do not. Children are more likely to repeat behaviour when they are praised, and less likely to repeat it when they are punished. This explanation is called behaviourist theory.

Behavouist theory, see page 197

> **Word check**
>
> **social learning theory** – the theory that people learn ways of behaving by copying others.

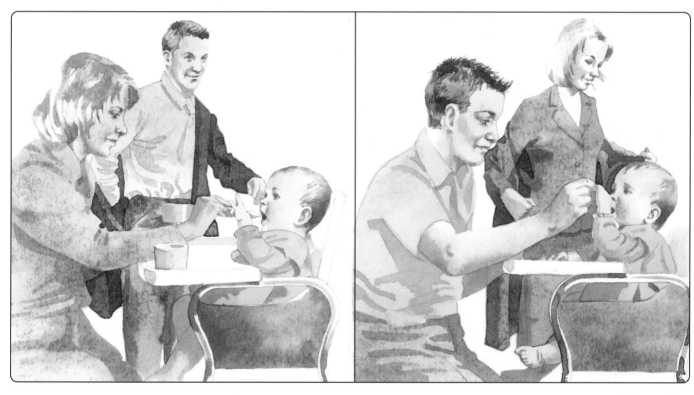

Role models

Learning about gender starts very early in infancy. An experiment took place to find out about gender. People were given the same baby to mind. Sometimes the baby was dressed in pink, and sometimes in blue. When the baby was dressed in blue, the people in the experiment assumed it was a boy, and said things like 'what a big, strong boy'. When the baby was dressed in pink, they assumed it was a girl, and said things like 'what a pretty girl'. They gave the baby dolls to play with when it was dressed in pink. When it was dressed in blue, they gave the baby toy cars. The experiment seemed to show that even before they can speak, infants are trained to behave in certain ways according to their sex. They are also encouraged to believe certain things about them are important, according to their gender, such as girls are pretty and boys are strong. What is happening is that the children are being taught that they should believe certain things about themselves because of their sex.

42 How do we learn about gender?

Effect of gender, see page 205

Turn back to page 205 of this unit to remind yourself how gender roles can be reinforced in education. Gender influences the development of self-concept and what children learn in this way affects their lives in adulthood.

The idea that children learn by watching is particularly important if young children are exposed to violence in the home. If they see their father beating their mother, for instance, they may grow up to believe that this is the way that a man should behave. Then they may repeat this behaviour when they have families of their own.

The effect of gender on adult behaviour

Adults are also affected by gender. Once there were clear gender roles. Men went out to work and earned the money, and women stayed at home and cared for the children and the home.

Today, people have more choice and it is not so easy to be exact when defining gender roles. Some women do stay at home and look after children, but they may think that this is not valued. Some believe that they are looked down upon by women who work. Some women who have careers have a positive self-concept of themselves as working women, but others feel guilty that they are not spending more time with their children.

Men are also affected by changes in gender roles. Some men want to play a greater part in caring for their children and some are happy to stay at home full-time to do so. Others think that an important part of being a man is to be the breadwinner. They may find their self-concept threatened if their partner earns more than they do.

Our self-concept, therefore, is influenced by the attitudes of those living around us. If we do not **conform** to these attitudes, views and opinions we may feel that we are not as good as others. We may be unhappy because we are not following what is accepted practice. This will affect our self-concept, the internal picture we have of ourselves.

Word check

conform – to act or behave in the same way as the rest of a group.

Culture

Word check

personal modesty – being reserved about exposing your body and in your sexual behaviour.

morality – conforming to accepted standards of conduct in society.

Culture is shared beliefs, customs and values. It includes things such as language, religion and other faiths, diet, dress, sport and music. It also includes ideas about things like **personal modesty**, **morality** and gender roles. Culture binds societies together. It gives people a shared identity and a sense of belonging. This is why it is important for someone's self-concept.

 How does culture affect self-concept?

A person's self-concept can be affected if health and social services are not provided in a way that is appropriate for them. They may not find information about services in their preferred language. Their dietary needs may not be met, or their ideas about personal modesty may be ignored. They may feel that the people providing the services do not think that they are important or valuable.

These attitudes may affect a person's self-concept. Their image of themselves may contribute to having a low self-esteem. They may feel angry that no-one has made the effort to find out what they want or what is best for them. They may become aggressive in order to draw attention to the real 'me'.

Kaz

Kaz is 76. He lives in a residential home. He is not able to eat the food provided because of his faith. Kaz needs a place set aside for him to pray several times each day and where he can follow the needs of his faith, but no one has responded to his request for this.

Kaz has become angry because of the discrimination. He has started shouting at other residents and at some of the care staff. He also cries a lot.

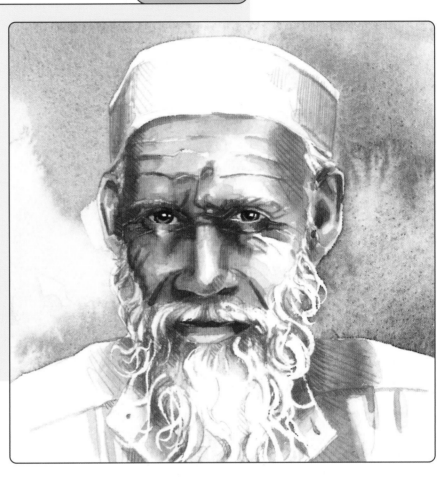

Kaz does not feel his needs are being met

Kaz

A1 Explain how the residential home could meet Kaz's cultural needs.

A2 How is Kaz's self-concept likely to be affected by the discrimination?

Key learning activity

K1 Explain how the discrimination could affect Kaz's relationship with the other residents.

K2 Explain the likely affect on Kaz's self-concept if the care workers were to meet his cultural needs.

Emotional development

Emotional development is very important to self-concept because it determines how we think about ourselves, and what we believe others think about us. Good emotional development and its effect on self-concept start almost from birth. The way in which parents discipline an infant will affect the infant's emotional development and self-concept.

Consider these different ways of disciplining children.

Carer A tries not to punish a young child unless it is absolutely necessary. When the child is doing something dangerous or naughty, the carer distracts them by offering them something interesting to do. When the child does something good, they are praised and rewarded. The child is often praised, and learns to do things because it feels good. If they are often praised, children develop a sense of themselves as valuable people who deserve respect.

Carer B shouts at their children and sometimes hits them when they do something the carer thinks is wrong. The children are often criticised and told they are naughty, or a nuisance. They are never praised for things they do well. They do not feel good about themselves because they are never told that they are good, but they are often told that they are bad. They do what they are told because they are afraid of being punished if they do not. The emotions they are learning are fear, guilt and anxiety.

44 How can a positive self-concept be developed in infants and children?

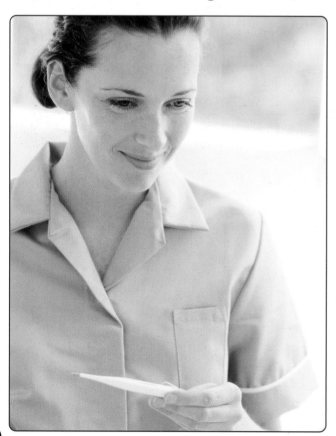

Someone who has had a positive experience in their emotional development has a strong self-concept. If someone is confident that they are valuable, then they believe in themselves and do not depend on other people's approval. They have confidence in everything they do, whether it is sitting an examination, asking someone out, or applying for a job. They can accept that sometimes things go wrong, and it is not necessarily their fault. When they are criticised, they can accept it if it is justified, and learn from it. They are optimistic about life. They present themselves confidently and have a realistic view of their abilities.

Someone with poor emotional development has a negative self-concept. They feel anxious about taking risks. This may make them shy and self-conscious. They may find it difficult to make friends because they are not sure what they have to offer.

They can be afraid of confrontation with others because they are not confident in their own opinions. They may put themselves down. They may be unable to react positively to criticism and either resent it or see it as a personal attack. They do not have a very good opinion about life and undervalue their abilities.

Full of confidence

Education

Educational experiences can have a major influence on self-concept. The way children are treated by their teachers and the relationships children form with other pupils can affect self-image. This is not only in childhood but throughout adolescence and adulthood as well. If children are encouraged in what they do well, they gain confidence and achieve more than if they are criticised for what they do poorly. Educational achievement is a positive influence on self-concept because it makes us feel good about ourselves.

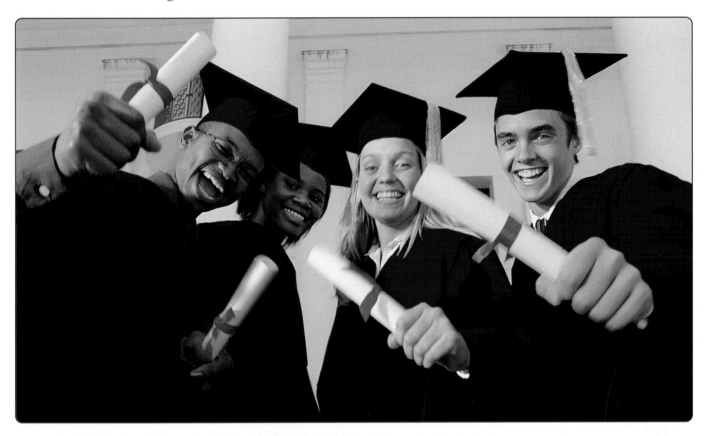

Academic success makes us feel good

Relationships with others

An important part of a person's self-concept is what they believe others think about them. Communication is an important part of all relationships. Good communication skills can help us to form positive relationships. It is in relationships that individuals find out what others think about them. If an individual has a trusting and honest relationship with another person, such as a friend, they may learn from them that others have a higher opinion of them than they thought. This will improve their self-esteem.

If, on the other hand, a person has poor relationships, particularly within their family, they may lack confidence and probably feel that they are not loved or valued. This could result in them being unable to form lasting relationships in adolescence and adulthood.

45 Why is a person who has experienced poor family relationships likely to have a poor self-concept?

Sexual orientation

Our sexual orientation is determined by whether we are attracted to members of the opposite or the same sex. Sexual orientation is an important part of self-concept.

Life experiences

Life experiences are the everyday things that happen to us. A single life experience is not likely to affect our self-concept, but life events when considered altogether can.

Infants and children

Infants' life experiences are very limited. Carers are responsible for all the life experiences of babies. These life experiences are very important for the development of a baby's self-concept.

As children get older their physical and intellectual development means that they can do more things for themselves. Their emotional and social development means that they can do things separately from their carers without getting distressed.

They start to make relationships with other people and their life experiences widen. Their self-concept is affected by other relationships, with teachers and friends, for example.

Adolescents

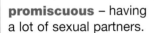

Word check

promiscuous – having a lot of sexual partners.

Adolescents become increasingly independent and their experiences widen. Most teenagers go through a period of rebellion. Usually parents can put up with this, and the rows and arguments pass. They are left with a good relationship. If adolescents have a bad relationship with their parents, they are more likely to turn to crime, drugs or alcohol abuse. They may become **promiscuous**. This can mean a young girl having an unwanted pregnancy. It increases the chances of sexually transmitted diseases being passed on. All these things limit opportunities and have a negative effect on self-concept.

Adults

Adults' life experiences are wider still as they become completely independent. They become workers and set up home for themselves. If their experience of work is satisfying, and they have a satisfactory relationship with their partner, then these are positive factors contributing to their self-concept. Sometimes these factors are not positive. They may experience bullying in the workplace or within a relationship. They may experience discrimination in their lives, because of their sex, sexuality, race or disability. All of these things can negatively affect self-concept.

Many older adults have very positive life experiences. They have good relationships with their families, and enjoy busy, active lives. However, older people can feel devalued by others, which has a negative effect on their self-concept.

Heather

CASE STUDY

Heather is in her early seventies. She is very active. She is a member of the Women's Institute, helps with many activities at her local church and plays bingo with her friends twice each week.

Every other weekend she either takes the train to Oxford to stay with her daughter and family or the family come to visit her. They all get on very well. Heather and her son-in-law, Simon can often be found laughing together. Simon cuts the grass for Heather when he visits as he thinks the machine is too heavy for her.

The whole family enjoys walks together and they go shopping at the weekend. Sometimes they go to the cinema. Heather likes being with her grandchildren and joins in some of the board games they play. She tries to go to their school plays and to any special events, like the Christmas Carol service.

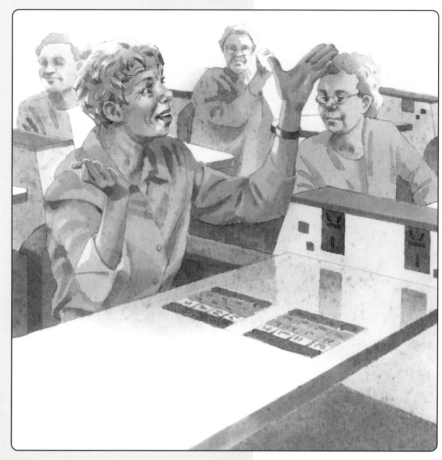

Heather enjoys playing bingo

C1 How is visiting their grandmother regularly and sharing activities and interests together likely to affect the self-concept of the grandchildren?

C2 What factors are influencing Heather's self-concept?

C3 How might Heather's self-concept be affected if her daughter and her family suddenly stopped visiting?

Key learning activity

ACTIVITY

K1 Explain what could contribute to having a poor self-concept in older adulthood.

K2 How can educational experiences affect a person's self-concept?

K3 How can gender affect self-concept?

The effects of life events on personal development

Getting started

How can life events affect an individual's personal development?

Life events are expected or unexpected experiences that can have a major effect on personal development. Some life events are expected. This means that we can be almost certain that they will happen to us, for example, starting school around the age of five. Everybody goes through physical changes such as puberty. We all eventually die, so this is expected!

Other life events are unexpected. This means they take us by surprise, and we have no way of knowing when or if they might happen. An example of this is a serious road accident. In this section we will learn about:

- relationship changes
- physical changes
- changes in life circumstances
- the effects that expected and unexpected life events can have on personal development
- how we adapt and use sources of support to cope with life events
- sources of support, for example, partners, family, friends, professional care services, voluntary and faith-based services.

An important life event

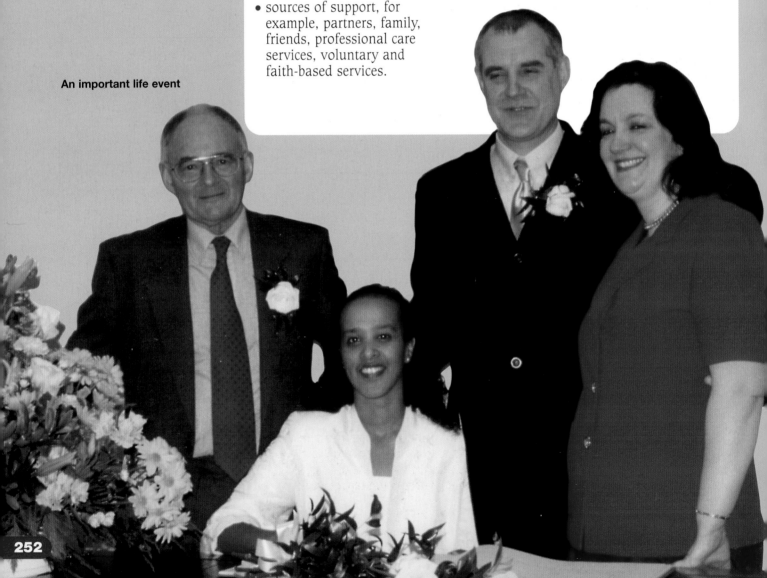

All life events provide the opportunity for personal growth.

They can also cause stress, which can have emotional effects such as anxiety and depression. We may have to make changes so that we can live comfortably with the new circumstances. Such changes promote personal development because what we learn from the experiences contributes to our personal development.

Events are on some occasions **expected** life events, but for other people the same event could be **unexpected**. For example, a birth in a family may be expected, if the partners have planned the pregnancy. For another couple, the birth might not have been planned and so it is unexpected.

46 What is the difference between expected and unexpected experience of life events?

Word check ✓

expected – something you know is going to happen; planned.

Word check ✓

unexpected – a surprise, not planned.

Relationship changes

Many of the most stressful life events are to do with relationship changes. These are often the most difficult to adapt to. Relationship changes include marriage, divorce and the death of a friend or partner.

Marriage

When two people get married, they enter into a contract. They promise to:

- be faithful to each other, which means that they will not have other sexual partners

- look after each other, by caring for each other physically if unwell, and by providing for each other financially

- share the responsibility for any children that they have together.

Some couples live together without getting married, but as 'partners'. They may have children. They may decide to get married at a later date or they may not. When two people decide to live together they have to make changes about the way they do routine tasks just as in a marriage. If one person insisted on having their own way all of the time the partnership would not work and there would be a breakdown in the relationship.

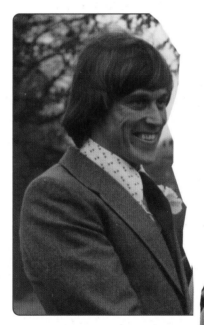
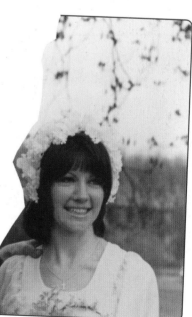

Marriage does not always last

Today divorce is common, but it still has a major impact on people's personal development. Losing a partner through divorce or separation can have many of the same social and emotional effects as bereavement – a sense of loss, grief, perhaps loneliness. There are also other effects; divorce often leaves both partners worse off financially.

The effect of divorce on the family

Divorce has many effects on the development of family members, especially children. One partner has to leave the home after divorce. The parent that stays behind is usually the one that has the main responsibility for the children. If they have no partner to help care for the children, they may have to give up work. If they cannot afford to stay in the house, they have all the extra problems of moving house.

It is often more stressful to bring up children alone. Children often stay with their mother when parents separate. Many fathers have access to children for a weekend, for example. This affects the personal development of both the children and their parents. Children may lack a role model. They may have difficulty in adjusting when their parents meet new partners. For some children, the completion of the divorce brings relief. It may mean the end of arguments and tension within the home.

47 How can divorce have a positive affect on development?

Living with a partner

More and more couples live together and do not get married at all.

This means that when buying or renting a house or buying furniture or other items, care has to be taken to sort out the legal aspects, for example, ownership of the goods. If the partnership breaks down, knowing who owns what may prevent quarrels and arguments.

If the couple have a child they have to decide whose surname the child will have.

As with marriage, partnerships can have a very positive effect on personal relationships. The two people learn to share and to communicate with one another. They have someone to talk to when problems occur and someone to share happy events.

48 How is living with a partner likely to affect development?

Birth in the family

For a young child the birth of a sibling can often be a **traumatic** life event. A first child is used to having all their parents' attention. When the new baby arrives, they have to adjust to having less attention. If they are well prepared for the new baby, made to feel important and reassured that they are still loved, then it can be a very positive experience. If they are not prepared for the new arrival, they can often be jealous.

Word check

traumatic – deep shock or upset.

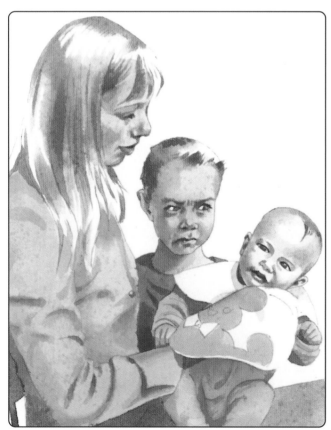

"I don't want him here."

The experience of having a new baby brother or sister could affect a child's development during adolescence and adulthood. It could mean that the eldest child always wants to be first, always wants to lead, because they feel that they will be pushed out or ignored if they are not seen to be the leader. Or it could mean that the person becomes withdrawn and feels guilty because they think they were not good enough, not valued.

A good experience of having brothers and sisters can result in developing a positive sense of our own worth. It means being able to share and enjoy being with others. We feel we do not always have to be first and can give support when required, or take the lead when necessary. Our development will be balanced.

49 How can the arrival of a sibling have a negative affect on the development of a previous only child?

Death of a friend or relative

The most difficult common life event to deal with is the death of a partner or of one's own child. Bereavement has physical, intellectual, emotional and social effects. The loss of a parent is something most of us experience, and the adjustment required depends on our life stage when it happens. While bereavement is a serious life event for an adult, it can be much more stressful for a child.

Grief is normal and a necessary response to the death of someone we love. Sometimes grief can last a long time; on other occasions it will be short-lived. Grief has several stages:

- shock and disbelief
- denial
- growing awareness of the loss
- acceptance of the loss.

It is important that people are allowed to work through their feelings and to give the bereaved person as much support as possible. If a person does not work through their grief they can develop feelings of guilt, blaming themselves for the death. This could lead to them feeling angry, resentful and to a sense of loneliness. They may become depressed or they could possibly become aggressive.

50 What are the stages of grief?

Carol and Brian　　　　　　　CASE STUDY

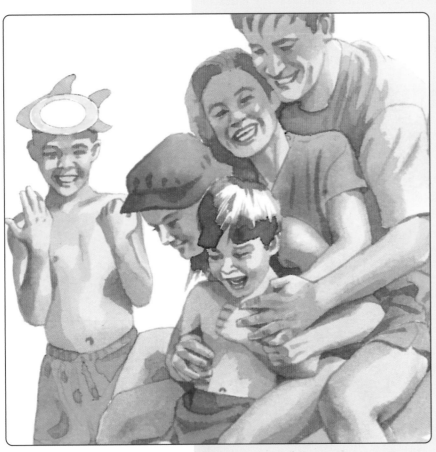

Carol and her partner, Brian have three children. All are healthy and appear to be happy. Christopher, the youngest child appears to have a cold, but soon he develops a fever. Purple spots appear and Christopher cannot bear any light near his eyes. His parents become quite worried and call the GP.

The GP immediately arranges for Christopher to be admitted to hospital. He is given a great deal of medical help, but unfortunately he dies. The doctors tell his parents that the cause of death is meningitis.

Carol and Brian with their family in happier times

C1 How are the parents likely to express their grief?

C2 How is the loss of a child likely to affect the development of the parents?

Key learning activity　　　　　ACTIVITY

K1 List THREE relationship changes that could occur as life events.

K2 For each relationship change given in K1 describe how the change could affect the development of an individual.

K3 Explain how divorce could have both a positive and negative affect on personal development.

Physical changes

Puberty

Puberty is a time of physical and emotional changes. It is the stage between childhood and adulthood, the attainment of sexual maturity. Both boys and girls experience puberty. There are changes in body size and shape. The reproductive organs start to function. Concern about appearance can sometimes lead to a lowering of self-confidence in teenagers.

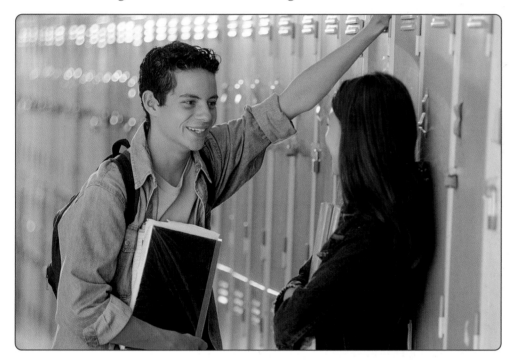

Adolescence is a time of change

Accident or injury

Becoming physically disabled through accident, injury or illness is a major life event. It is usually unexpected. A person who becomes disabled has to adapt their lifestyle, depending on the degree of disability. They may lose some independence and have to rely on others for daily living tasks that they were once able to do for themselves. An extreme example is someone who becomes completely paralysed and requires help with all their bodily functions. A problem that many people have to face in adapting to disability is the prejudice of others. Those with disabilities often complain that they are treated like children; people tend to speak to their carers rather than to them. This makes the person who is not able-bodied feel inferior, as though they do not count. It is almost as though they are not present in the conversation.

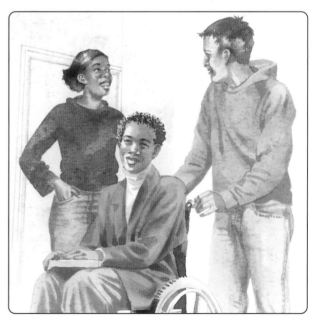

Being ignored by others can be damaging

Becoming disabled may result in losing a job and having to retrain. It may involve a loss of income, or moving to more appropriate accommodation. It may also require changes in hobbies or interests.

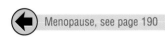
Menopause, see page 190

The menopause

The menopause signals the end of a woman's reproductive life. She may have to come to terms with the fact that she can no longer have children. Turn back to page 190 to remind yourself about what happens at this stage of development.

51 Why might a woman feel a sense of loss when the menopause occurs?

Changes in life circumstances

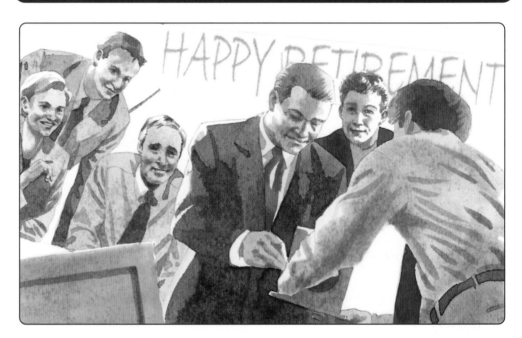

Retirement is a major life event

All changes in life circumstances have some common features. The most important is that they involve changes in existing relationships, and a need to develop new ones. Moving house, changing schools and changing or losing a job all mean leaving some relationships behind – neighbours, friends, teachers, bosses and colleagues. To adapt successfully to the change, we must make new relationships, sometimes in a new role.

Moving house or away from home

When someone moves house or moves away to start a new job or college, they leave behind familiar friends, neighbours and neighbourhoods. Leaving friends and neighbours matters because you lose the physical, emotional and social support they offer. Life is much easier with these networks to help. Parents, for instance, have to know who they can trust to babysit for them. Good neighbours can help in all sorts of ways, for instance by watching the house when we are away on holiday, or helping when we are ill. When we move house we have to build new relationships.

Maria

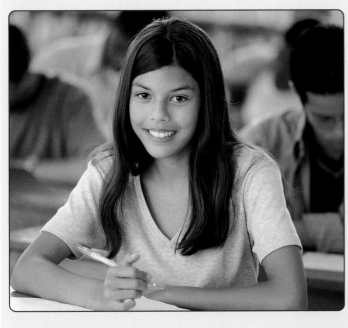

Maria

Maria has been successful in her examinations. She is moving away from home to go to college to study health and beauty. She has lived with her family in a rural area all her life. None of her friends are going to the same college and she is sure she will miss them.

At college Maria will be sharing a house with three other girls she has not met before. She is very nervous and anxious about the move, but it is something that she wants to do.

Maria ACTIVITY

A1 Describe the difficulties Maria might have to cope with when she moves to college.

A2 List FOUR ways Maria could help to prepare herself for the move.

A3 Explain how Maria's development is likely to be affected by moving away from home.

Key learning activity

K1 If Maria had an accident that affected her ability to walk how might her development be affected?

K2 How is Maria's leaving home to go to college likely to affect her parents' development?

Starting school

Starting school may be the first time that a child has been away from their main carer for a whole day. The child has to become more independent and make relationships with other children. This can be quite a frightening experience if the child is not properly prepared. Parents who have previously been close at hand are no longer available. Relationships with new adults and new children are formed. Rules must be followed. All these changes can have a negative effect on the child's development.

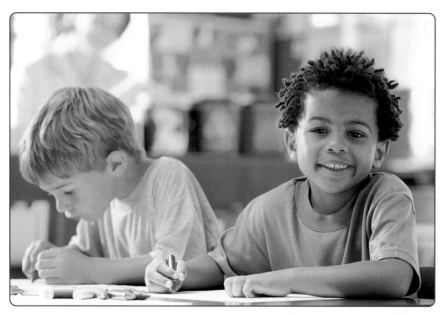

A well-prepared child settles happily into school

A child may become very 'clingy' to the parent and make a fuss when it is the time for them to leave. They may become withdrawn and sit in a corner away from the other children, refusing to join in the activities. The child may behave like this because they do not understand what is happening. They may think they have been abandoned or that they are being punished. This may lead to the child having nightmares or bedwetting. They may become aggressive towards their parents. It could lead to the child disliking school and underachieving in their work.

A child who is well prepared before starting school is more likely to enjoy a positive experience.

52 Why is it important to prepare a child for starting school?

Starting work

Starting work involves intellectual development in learning what the job involves. New skills and knowledge have to be acquired. Emotional developments also take place when starting work. This is particularly true if working in the health, social care or early years sector. For example, as a carer, if you are working with someone who is rude and bad-tempered, or very slow, you have to deal with your anger or impatience in a mature way.

At work we meet new colleagues and have the opportunity to make more friends. Our social development is therefore affected.

As working means earning money, we become financially independent. This means that we may no longer be dependent on parents for money. We have to learn how to manage our finances. This is an intellectual development.

Work may be physically challenging and this affects our physical development.

Starting work is usually considered an expected life event as most people at some time have to earn their living. If we like the work we do we will be mentally stimulated and happy, with a sense of fulfilment and well-being. Work can give a positive direction to our lives.

During our adult lives we are likely to spend many hours at work. If we do not like the work we do we could become depressed and physically ill. Many people today suffer from stress as a result of work. This could be because they are asked to do too much. They may find the work too difficult or perhaps the work does not suit them. Whatever the reason, the negative effects can make a person feel that they are a failure.

53 Why is it important to like the work we do?

Retirement

Retirement is when we stop working altogether. We may get an occupational pension. We may be at an age where a state pension can be claimed. What we do for a living is an important part of our identity. When we retire, we lose the physical, intellectual, emotional and social stimulation provided by work. Some people are unhappy when their working lives come to an end. Others are very happy. Whether retirement is a positive or negative development depends upon how people deal with it. People who are happy to retire are those who find other ways of getting the stimulation that they used to get from work.

54 Why can retirement have a negative affect on development?

Redundancy and unemployment

Unlike retirement, redundancy and unemployment are often unexpected life events. Unemployment means not having a job. Redundancy means losing your job because the job has disappeared, perhaps because a company has closed down.

Like retirement, unemployment and redundancy mean losing physical, intellectual, emotional and social stimulation provided by work. Redundancy is different from retirement because it often happens unexpectedly. It can affect development because people worry about how they are going to manage financially. Too much worry can make us ill, both physically and mentally, through stress.

Some people who are made redundant, particularly older workers, find it very difficult to get another job before they reach retirement age. This may make them feel undervalued and lose confidence in themselves.

55 What is the difference between retirement and redundancy?

Many people who are unemployed feel bored because they do not have enough to do to fill their time. They become depressed if working is very important to their sense of identity. They may find their relationship with their partner suffers. This can be especially true for men who are used to providing for their family. They may find it very difficult to be dependent on their partner or on benefits.

56 How can unemployment affect development?

Life events do not come along one at a time. One life event may be related to several others. For instance, someone who is in a relationship and has children is offered a promotion at work that involves moving house. They may have to learn new skills, and their partner may have to give up their own job, too. The children have to change schools, and everyone in the family leaves friends behind in the move.

Sources of support

Partners, family and friends

Partners, family and friends are often called informal carers. They can help by providing physical, emotional and social support to make it possible for us to cope with the effects of life events.

By talking about our problems with others, they can appear to be smaller than we thought. Sometimes, talking to someone can bring clarity to the situation.

They may offer us practical support such as cooking, washing or housework if we are unable to do things for ourselves. This support may be short term – for example, someone who has had a baby often welcomes help after the birth. Friends may help out when we are ill.

Informal carers also give emotional support. Friends are important to us because we know that they will listen to our problems. They will understand why we are upset. Social support is also important. For example, after a divorce or bereavement we can feel lonely and isolated. Friends may visit and encourage us to go out. This is very important for meeting new people and rebuilding our lives.

57 Who are informal carers?

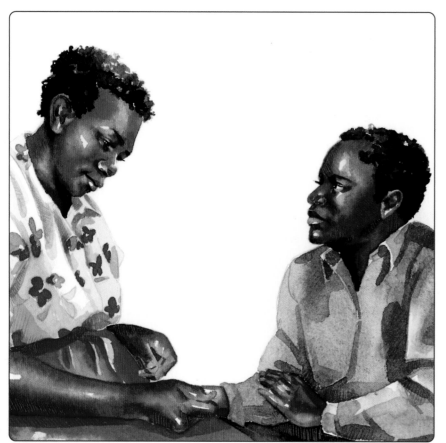

A friend can help

How can we, as informal carers, help people to cope with life events? We can help by:

- being available
- not being anxious or upset but by being concerned
- listening when a person wants to talk and not interrupting
- giving reassurance
- offering to share a meal with the person occasionally
- not changing the subject when a person wants to talk about their problem.

Making practical suggestions is particularly helpful as the person can then do something positive to help.

58 How can informal carers help people cope with change?

Professional care workers and services

Professional carers are people who are paid to look after us when we need help, particularly when a life event has changed our lives.

Examples of professionals who provide help are:

- home care assistant – helps with shopping, cleaning and preparing meals

- GP – gives medical checks, listens, gives advice and writes prescriptions

- social worker – assesses a client's needs

- occupational therapist – assesses how a client's home needs to be adapted.

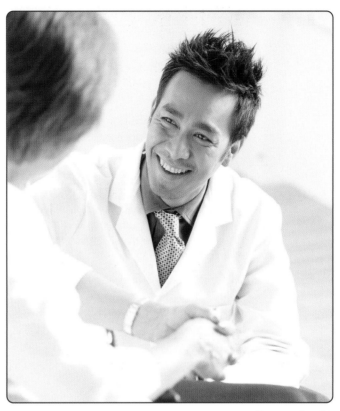

Care professional providing support

59 Can you think of others who could provide support for a person who is trying to cope with a life event?

60 What is the difference between an informal and a professional carer?

Voluntary and faith-based services

Many voluntary organisations provide information, support and services to help people cope with the effects of life events, such as:

- Citizens Advice Bureau – refers people to specialist organisations

- National Childbirth Trust – helps people to prepare for parenthood

- Relate – helps couples who are having relationship/marriage problems

- CRUSE – helps people who have suffered a bereavement.

Many people get help from their faith (religious belief) when they experience life events, especially when they are bereaved. Having a faith can give emotional and social support. Priests, clerics, other religious workers and volunteers can be very important. They can give advice and comfort during times of personal crisis and other life events.

61 How can having a faith or belief help us to cope with life events?

Without help during life event changes, some people are unable to cope. The life event may have a major effect on their personal development. The result may be that they have very low self-esteem, become depressed or even suicidal. They may need medication to help them manage depression or to sleep. Without help the situation could get worse. We all need to remember that we may need help when life events overtake us. We should not be afraid of asking for that help.

Gary CASE STUDY

Gary has a wife and a daughter, aged six. He has been working in a car factory for 15 years, earning good money. The family lives near the factory in their own semi-detached house that Gary is buying on a mortgage. The family are reasonably well-off.

Without very much notice Gary is told that the factory is to be closed. The cars are to be built in another part of the country. Gary is not offered a job in the new factory, but made redundant.

Gary tries to get another job, but so many other people want jobs, too. He applies for 78 and does not get any of them. He becomes depressed. Money is running out and arguments break out between Gary and his wife. The atmosphere gets so bad that Gary just goes out and walks around each day. He starts going into the pub when he gets his dole money and drinks so much that there is no money left for food.

His wife decides that she cannot put up with the situation any longer, so she leaves Gary. She goes back to her mother and takes their little girl with her.

Gary continues to drink. He does not pay the mortgage on the house or the bills. Eventually the house is re-possessed by the mortgage company, leaving Gary homeless. He has lost everything!

Redundancy ACTIVITY

A1 Explain what is meant by 'being made redundant'.

A2 How do you think that being made redundant affected Gary's emotional and social development?

A3 When Gary was made redundant which voluntary service could he have visited to get support? How would this service have provided help?

A4 How could family and friends have helped Gary when he was made redundant?

A5 Explain the affect Gary's redundancy might have had on his wife's personal development.

 ## Key learning activity

K1 How can faith-based organisations help people cope with life changes?

K2 Gary had a child of six. How would the child's personal development be affected by the changes in the family circumstances?

K3 What professional support could have helped Gary cope with the changes in his life?

• Explain how each service would help.

Appendix

Appendix 1 – Daily recommended vitamin intake (mg)

Nutrients	Babies	Children	Men 19–65	Men over 65	Women 19–55	Women over 55
Vitamin A Retinol	0.35	0.5	0.75	0.75	0.75	0.75
Vitamin B1 Thiamine	0.2	0.7	1.1	0.9	0.8	0.7
Vitamin B2 Riboflavin			1.7	1.5	1.2	1.0
Niacin Nicotinamide			20	17	14	12
Vitamin B6 Pyridoxine			2	1.5	1.4	1.1
Folic acid	50	100	200	200	200	200
Vitamin B12 Cyanocobalamin	0.3	0.8	2	2	2	2
Vitamin C Ascorbic acid	25	30	40	40	50	50
Vitamin D	8.5					
Vitamin E Tocopherols			10	10	7	7

Appendix 2 – Daily recommended mineral intake (mg)

Nutrient	Babies	Children	Men 19–65	Men over 65	Women 19–55	Women over 55
Calcium	525	450	800	800	800	1000
Iodine			150	150	120	120
Iron	1.7	6.1	7	7	12.6	5.7
Magnesium	55	120	320	320	270	270
Phosphorus	400	350	1000	1000	1000	1000
Potassium	800	1100	3500	3500	3500	3500
Sodium	210	700	1600	1600	1600	1600
Zinc			12	12	12	12

Appendix 3 – Energy values

1g carbohydrates:	4 Calories/16.8 kilojoules
1g protein:	4 Calories/16.8 kilojoules
1g fat:	9 Calories/37.8 kilojoules

Appendix 4 – Calorie counter

Food	Measure	Calories
Milk (full cream)	1 cup	167
Milk (skimmed)	1 cup	88
Milk (soya)	1 cup	160
Yogurt (natural)	200g	160
Yogurt (low fat)	200g	120
Yogurt (flavoured)	200g	190
Cheese	30g	120
Cheese (grated)	1/2 cup	240
Ice cream (single flavour)	1 scoop	90
Butter	1 tsp	36
Margarine	1 tsp	36
Oil (vegetable, etc.)	1 tbsp	176
Egg (large)	67g	100
Corned beef	100g	210
Beef (fillet steak)	100g	196
Beef (rump steak)	100g	190
Beef (T Bone steak)	100g	135
Beef (minced)	100g	210
Leg of lamb (roast)	2 slices	170
Bacon (grilled)	1 rasher	112
Chicken (roasted breast)	100g	110
Chicken (leg/thigh)	100g	210
Fish (white fish, low fat)	100g	100
Baked beans	220g	205
Bread (white plain)	1 slice	66
Bread (wholemeal)	1 slice	62
Rice (white, cooked)	1/2 cup	92
Rice (brown, cooked)	1/2 cup	93
Biscuit (chocolate chip)	1	35
Biscuit (chocolate)	1	98
Biscuit (ginger)	1	42
Chocolate (plain/nut/fruit)	5–6 rows	160
Almonds	25–30	170
Cashews	12–16	180
Hazelnuts	30g	185
Peanuts (raw)	30g	120
Apple (medium)	1	65

Food	Measure	Calories
Apricot (medium)	1	15
Banana (medium)	1	87
Grapefruit (medium)	1/2	20
Grapes	125g	125
Kiwi fruit (medium)	1	40
Lemon	1	23
Mango	1	102
Orange (medium)	1	80
Peach	1	40
Pear	1	69
Pineapple	1 slice	33
Plum	1	33
Melon	1/2 med	135
Strawberries	6 med	10
Tomato	1 med	20
Dried apple rings	10 rings	75
Dried apricots	5–6	80
Dried banana chips	1/4 cup	155
Dates	4–5	83
Prunes (moist)	2–3	70
Sultanas	2 tbsp	92
Bean sprouts	100g	30
Asparagus spears	3 med	10
Beans	1/2 cup	13
Broccoli	2 florets	11
Cabbage	1/2	7
Carrots	1 small	23
Cauliflower	1/2 cup	20
Cucumber	150g	12
Lettuce	3 leaves	2
Lentils (cooked)	100g	260
Mushrooms	1/2 cup	15
Onions	medium	30
Peas	1/4 cup	20
Potato	medium	105
Lemonade	375ml	160
Tonic water	375ml	135

Appendix 5 – Calorie controlled menus

The following menus each contain between 1500 and 1800 Calories.
You can use these as a guide when planning your own menus.

Menu 1

Breakfast
1/2 cup orange juice
1 cup cooked oatmeal
1 cup low fat milk

Lunch
3 slices (3 ounces) turkey breast
2 slices wholegrain bread
Fresh spinach leaves and tomato slices
1 tablespoon reduced fat mayonnaise
1 apple

Snack
1/2 cup tomato juice
2 large rice cakes

Dinner
1 cup black bean soup
1 corn tortilla
toasted and topped with 1 cup chopped cooked vegetables
and 1/2 cup grated reduced fat cheese
3 fresh pineapple rings, or tinned in fruit juice
1 cup sugar free, fat free fruit yoghurt

Menu 2

Breakfast
1 cup of melon cubes
1/2 cup bran flakes cereal
1 cup low fat milk

Lunch
1 cup lentil soup
Salad
1 cup raw spinach, 1 cup sliced mushrooms
1 tablespoon reduced fat salad dressing
2 large or 4 small bread sticks
1/2 cup low fat dip

Snack
1 cup grapes
1 slice (3/4 ounce) reduced fat cheese

Dinner
1 large white fish fillet grilled with 1 teaspoon olive oil
1 cup steamed broccoli spears
1/2 small baked potato topped with 1/2 cup non fat plain yoghurt
1/2 cup fruit salad

Snack
3 crackers
1 cup low fat milk

Menu 3

Breakfast
1/2 grapefruit
1 slice wholegrain toast
1 tablespoon reduced calorie margarine or butter
2 eggs, scrambled in a microwave oven
or non-stick pan without fat
1 cup low-fat milk

Lunch

Pasta salad
1 cup cooked pasta with 1 ounce reduced fat cheese cubes,
1/2 cup chopped cooked vegetables and 2 tablespoons
low fat salad dressing
1 cup melon chunks
2 bread sticks
1/2 cup vegetable or tomato juice

Dinner

3 ounces lean steak
sliced and wrapped in 2 tortillas with 1/2 cup diced tomato,
1 cup raw spinach leaves and 1/2 cup red or sweet white onion slices
1 kiwi, peeled and sliced

Snack

2 cups of microwave popcorn

Menu 4

Breakfast

3 small pancakes
with 2 tablespoons reduced calorie jam and 1 cup strawberries
1 cup low fat milk

Lunch

Tuna salad sandwich
2 slices wholegrain bread, 3 ounces tuna, chopped celery,
lettuce leaves, 1 tablespoon reduced fat mayonnaise
1 large pear or apple
2 large rice cakes

Dinner

1/2 chicken breast, baked or grilled with no skin
1/2 cup cooked brown rice
1 cup steamed aubergine and carrots
1 small roll
1 tablespoon reduced calorie margarine or butter
1 cup fat free, sugar free hot cocoa, made with low-fat milk
3 fat free biscuits

Menu 5

Breakfast

1 large bagel toasted with 1 ounce reduced fat soft cheese
1 cup strawberries

Lunch

1 cup split pea soup
1 wholewheat pitta pocket
filled with shredded lettuce, 1 ounce reduced fat feta cheese,
1/2 cup chopped tomato and 1 tablespoon reduced fat
vinaigrette dressing
1 peach or 1/2 cup canned peaches in unsweetened juice
2 gingersnaps

Dinner

3 ounces lean pork
stir-fried with 1/2-cup sweet red pepper, 1/2-cup onion
and 1/2 cup sliced mushrooms in 2 teaspoons vegetable oil
1/2 cup cooked brown rice
1 cup fresh pineapple cubes
or 1/2 cup canned pineapple in unsweetened juice
1/2 cup low fat frozen yoghurt

Appendix 6 – Sample of a healthy two-day diet plan

	Day 1	Day 2
	Total Calories around 1950	Total Calories: around 1975
	53% carbohydrate 18% protein 29% fat	52% carbohydrate 18% protein 30% fat
Breakfast	orange juice, peaches and yogurt oatmeal wholewheat toast with soft margarine and marmalade tea with low fat milk	banana Bran flakes cinnamon raisin toasted muffin with soft margarine coffee with low fat milk
Snack	fresh fruit	orange
Lunch	vegetable soup sandwich with turkey, lettuce, tomato, cheese and mayonnaise salad iced tea	grilled chicken Caesar salad sliced French bread with soft margarine peach crisp iced tea
Snack	frozen yogurt	apple
Dinner	baked pork chop with pineapple sauce pureed potato broccoli spears wholewheat roll with soft margarine iced tea	egg drop soup beef and broccoli stir fry over pasta or rice bread stick tea

Appendix 7 – The Hall-Jones scale

Class	Definition
1	Professional and high administrative
2	Managerial and executive
3	Inspectional, supervisory and other non-manual, higher grade
4	Inspectional, supervisory and other non-manual, lower grade
5	Skilled manual and routine grades of non-manual
6	Semi-skilled
7	Unskilled manual

Appendix 8 – Sexually transmitted infections

STI	What to watch for	How do you get this STI?	What can happen?
Chlamydia	• Symptoms usually appear 7–21 days after infection. Many women and some men have no symptoms. • Women: unusual discharge from the vagina; bleeding from the vagina between periods; burning or pain when you urinate; pain in abdomen; sometimes fever and nausea. • Men: watery or white discharge from the penis; burning or pain when you urinate; pain or swelling in the testicles.	• Vaginal or anal sex with someone who has chlamydia.	• YOU CAN GIVE CHLAMYDIA TO YOUR SEXUAL PARTNER(S). • Can lead to a more serious infection. • Reproductive organs can be damaged. • Fertility may be affected for both men and women. • A woman with chlamydia can give it to her baby during childbirth.
Genital herpes	• Symptoms usually appear 2–20 days after infection. • Some people have mild or no symptoms. Flu-like symptoms; small, painful blisters on the genitals (or mouth); itching or burning before the blisters appear.	• Vaginal, oral or anal sex or skin-to-skin contact with someone who has herpes. • Oral herpes can be transmitted to the genitals during oral sex. • Transmission without symptoms can occur.	• YOU CAN GIVE HERPES TO YOUR SEXUAL PARTNER(S) • Herpes symptoms can be treated, but an infected person will always have the virus. • A woman with herpes can give it to her baby during childbirth. • Symptoms may recur.
Gonorrhoea	• Symptoms usually appear 2–10 days after infection. Many people have no symptoms. • Women: thick, yellow or white discharge from the vagina; burning or pain when you urinate; more pain than usual during periods; cramps and pain in the lower abdomen. • Men: thick, yellow or white discharge from the penis; burning or pain when you urinate.	• Vaginal, oral or anal sex with someone who has gonorrhoea.	• YOU CAN GIVE GONORRHOEA TO YOUR SEXUAL PARTNER(S). • Can lead to more serious infection. • Reproductive organs can be damaged. • Fertility may be affected for both men and women. • A woman with gonorrhoea can give it to her baby during childbirth.

STI	What to watch for	How do you get this STI?	What can happen?
Hepatitis B	• Symptoms usually appear 2–6 months after infection. • Majority of those infected have no symptoms. • Fatigue and weakness; anorexia (loss of appetite); jaundice and darkened urine; nausea and vomiting; fever and abdominal pain.	• Vaginal, oral or anal sex with someone who has the virus (it is 100 times more infectious than HIV). • Sharing needles with someone who is infected. • Close contact with infected blood, semen, saliva or vaginal secretions.	• YOU CAN GIVE HEPATITIS B TO YOUR SEXUAL PARTNER(S). • You can develop a lifelong infection, chronic liver disease or liver cancer. • You can infect future children if you become a carrier.
HIV/AIDS (Human Immuno-Deficiency Virus)	• Symptoms appear several months to several years after infection. • Unexplained weight loss; persistent diarrhoea; swollen lymph glands; purple bumps on the skin and inside the mouth, nose and rectum; recurrent yeast infections.	• Anal, vaginal and, possibly, oral sex with someone who is infected with the virus. • Also spread by sharing needles (to inject drugs) with someone who is infected with the virus.	• YOU CAN GIVE HIV TO YOUR SEXUAL PARTNER(S) OR SOMEONE WITH WHOM YOU SHARE A NEEDLE. • HIV cannot be cured. Most people die from a disease linked with HIV infection. • A pregnant woman with the virus can pass it to her baby.
Genital warts	• Symptoms usually appear within 3-6 months after infection. • In some cases, symptoms may not appear for years. • Small, bumpy warts on the genitals and anus; the warts do not go away; itching or burning around the genitals.	• Vaginal, oral or anal sex or skin-to-skin contact with someone who has the virus. • Transmission without symptoms can happen (when no warts are visible).	• YOU CAN GIVE IT TO YOUR SEXUAL PARTNER(S). • Symptoms can be treated, but an infected person will always have the virus • More warts appear.
Syphilis	• First stage: symptoms usually appear 1–12 weeks after infection. A painless, reddish-brown sore/chancre on the mouth or genitals; chancre lasts 1–5 weeks; chancre heals. • Second stage: symptoms usually appear 2–6 weeks after chancre disappears. A rash anywhere on the body; flu-like feelings; rash and flu-like feelings go away. • Third stage: may not appear until several years after infection. Lesions of the skin appear; the heart muscle is affected, leading to heart attack; the nervous system is affected, possibly leading to dementia.	• Vaginal, oral or anal sex with someone who has syphilis.	• YOU CAN GIVE SYPHILIS TO YOUR SEXUAL PARTNER(S). • A pregnant woman with syphilis can pass it to her baby (in the uterus). • Can cause heart disease, brain damage, blindness and death.

Appendix 9 – Care values and principles of the early years sector

1 The welfare of the child

The welfare of the child is paramount. All early years workers must give precedence to the rights and well-being of the children they work with. Children should be listened to, and their opinions and concerns treated seriously. Management of children's behaviour should emphasise positive expectations for that behaviour, and responses to unwanted behaviour should be suited to the child's stage of development. A child must never be slapped, smacked, shaken, humiliated, belittled or isolated.

2 Keeping children safe and maintaining a healthy and safe environment

a Keeping children safe

Work practice should help prevent accidents to children and adults, and to protect their health. Emergency procedures of the work setting, including record keeping, must be adhered to. Every early years worker has a responsibility to:

- contribute to the protection of children from abuse and exploitation, according to her/his work role

- report any suspicions of abuse, neglect or ill treatment to their relevant line manager.

b Maintaining a healthy and safe working environment

Every individual, no matter what their work role, has a duty and responsibility to implement and maintain safe working practices and procedures, and to bring to the attention of others, practices that have not been observed.

3 Working in partnership with parents/families

Parents and families occupy a central position in their children's lives, and early years workers must never try to take over that role inappropriately. Parents and families should be listened to as experts on their own child/children. Information about children's development and progress should be shared openly with parents. Respect must be shown for families' traditions and child care practices, and every effort made to comply with parent's wishes for their children.

4 Children's learning and development

Children learn more and faster in their earliest years than at any other time in life. Development and learning in these earliest years lay the foundations for abilities, characteristics and skills in later life. Learning begins at birth (some research suggests before birth). The care and education of children are interwoven.

Children should be offered a range of experiences and activities that support all aspects of their development; social, physical, intellectual, linguistic, emotional, creative. The choice of experiences and activities (the 'curriculum') should depend on accurate assessment of the stage of development reached by the child, following observation and discussion with families. Early years workers have varying responsibilities concerning the planning and implementation of the curriculum, according to their work role, but all contributions to such planning and implementation should set high expectations for children and build on their achievements and interests. Child-initiated play and activities should be valued and recognised as well as the adult planned curriculum. Written records should be kept of children's progress, and these records should be shared with parents and used to inform planning.

5 Valuing diversity

Britain is a multi-racial, multi-cultural society. The contributions made to this society by a variety of cultural groups should be viewed in a positive light. Information about varying traditions, customs and festivals should be presented as a source of pleasure and enjoyment to all children including those in areas where there are few members of minority ethnic groups. Children should be helped to develop a sense of their identity within their racial, cultural and social groups as well as having the opportunity to learn about cultures different from their own. No one culture should be represented as superior to any other: pride in one's own cultural and social background does not require condemnation of that of other people.

6 Equality of opportunity

Each child should be offered equality of access to opportunities to learn and develop, and so work towards her/his potential. Each child is a unique individual; early years workers must respect this individuality. Children should not be treated 'all the same'. In order to meet a child's needs, it is necessary to treat each child 'with equal concern'. Some children need more and/or different support in order to have equality of opportunity. It is essential to avoid stereotyping children on the basis of gender, racial origins, cultural or social background (including religion, language, class and family pattern), or ability. Such stereotypes may act as barriers to equality of access to opportunity. Early years workers should demonstrate their valuing of children's racial and other personal characteristics in order to help them develop self-esteem.

These principles of equality of access to opportunity and avoidance of stereotyping must also be applied to interactions with adult family members, colleagues and other professionals. Any person who is responsible for the actions of others within their organisation/setting must ensure that equal opportunities are applied in all work activities, practices and procedures.

7 Anti-discrimination

Early years workers must not discriminate against any child, family or groups in society on the grounds of gender, racial origins, cultural or social background (including religion, language, class and family pattern), disability or sexuality. They must acknowledge and address any personal beliefs or opinions which prevent them respecting the value systems of other people. They must comply with legislation and the policies of their work setting relating to discrimination. Children learn prejudice from their earliest years, and must be provided with accurate information to help them avoid prejudice. Expressions of prejudice by children or adults must be challenged. Support must be offered to those children or adults who are the objects of prejudice and discrimination. Early years workers have a powerful role to play in nurturing greater harmony amongst various groups in our society for future generations.

8 Confidentiality

Information about children and families must never be shared with others, without the permission of the family. The only exception to this is where a child has been abused, or is at risk from abuse, when agreed guidelines must be followed. Early years workers must adhere to the policy of their work setting concerning confidential information, including passing information to colleagues. Information about other workers must also be handled in a confidential manner.

9 Working with others

a Working with other professionals

Advice and support should be sought from other professionals with prior parental agreement, in the best interests of children and families. Information should be shared with them, subject to the principles of confidentiality. Respect should be shown for the roles of other professionals.

b Working in partnership with others

It is important to take into consideration the thoughts, feelings and beliefs of others within the setting and from outside the setting. Valuing the comments and actions of others is essential to maintain harmony and reduce potential conflict. For those in a management/supervisory role treating all staff equally is imperative to ensure productive working relationships. Establishing the professional development needs of staff and helping them to meet these needs is important within this role.

10 The reflective practitioner

Early years workers should use any opportunity they are offered or which arises to reflect on their practice and principles. They should make use of the conclusions from such reflection in developing and extending their practice. Seeking advice and support to help resolve queries or problems should be seen as a form of strength and professionalism. Opportunities for in-service training and/or continuous professional development should be used to the maximum.

Within the reflective process it is essential that practitioners, whatever their work role, update their knowledge and understanding of current policy, legislation and practice, ensuring that policy is linked with practice.

Glossary

Abstinence – avoidance, not taking part in; saying no

Abuse – to hurt someone by taking advantage of their inability to protect themselves

Access – arrange to see

Acid rain – rain that is acidic due to mixing with sulphur dioxide gas pollution

Actively – being involved

Addiction – being dependent on something, for example drugs or alcohol

Adoption – accepting responsibility for a child who is not one's own

Adrenaline – a hormone that stimulates the body to be alert

Aerobic – using oxygen

Aggravate – make worse

Agility – being able, quick, nimble and active

Alcohol dependency – needing alcohol every day; not being able to do without alcohol

Aims – an overall plan

Amino acids – chemicals that are the building blocks of protein

Anaerobic – not using oxygen

Anorexia – illness where the sufferer does not eat to avoid putting on weight

Artery – a blood vessel that carries blood away from the heart

Arthritis – joint inflammation or infection

Asthma – lung disease that makes you short of breath

Aspect – a part or area

Assertiveness – being firm and confident

Assess – to work out or estimate

Assessment of need – a care worker making decisions about the health, social care or early years needs of a person

At risk – may be in danger

Attachment – forming a close relationship with someone

Attitude – thoughts, views and behaviour

Balance – in the correct proportions

Barrier – something that stops a person doing something

Behaviourist theory – the theory that people learn the ways of behaving through rewards and punishments

Bereavement – losing someone close to you or well known to you

Biologically – how we function as human animals

Bisexual – someone who has sexual relationships with both male and female partners

Body Mass Index (BMI) – a scientific calculation that gives an index number that relates to a person's size

Bonding – forming a very close link/emotional attachment

Braille – a method of reading by running fingers over raised symbols

Breast screening – checking the breasts for signs of cancer

Bronchitis – inflammation of the small airways of the lungs

Bubonic plague – a killer disease that was active in the Middle Ages

Budget – an amount of money put aside for a certain purpose

Bulimia – disorder where people make themselves vomit in order to keep their weight down

Bulk – the biggest part

Calorie – unit of energy

Campaign – activity to promote an issue or product

Carbon monoxide – poisonous gas

Carcinogen – substance that can cause cancer

Cardio-vascular – relating to heart and blood vessels

Care need – requiring the services of health or social care or early years

Care setting – a place where people are cared for or looked after

Carrier – having one defective gene but appearing to be normal

Category – class or group

Cervical smear – testing the neck of the uterus for signs of cancer

Challenge – a problem, something that is difficult

Chart – document containing values and measurements

Chicken pox – a disease that affects mostly children, giving them spots and a fever

Cholesterol – fatty substance needed by the body and carried in the blood

Chronic – constant or continuing for a long time

Circulation – movement of blood around the body

Circumstances – the situation a person is in

Cirrhosis – a disease that damages the liver, can be caused by alcohol

Client – a person who has a need and is helped by a trained person

Code of practice – a set of guidelines; a framework within which to work

Cognitive – to do with thinking

Cold turkey – phase that drug addicts go through when they give up drugs; withdrawal symptoms

Colleague – person you work with

Common – shared by two or more people

Communicate – transfer information between two individuals

Community – group of people living in the same area, or having something in common

Community care – supporting people in their own homes

Community services – help for local people who have health or social or early years needs but who wish to remain in their own homes

Community trust – primary care groups and trust hospitals joining together to provide services

Companionship – having someone around to keep you from getting lonely

Complex – difficult, or having many functions

Component – a part of

Concept – the way we organise information in our minds; an abstract idea

Confidentiality – keeping information to oneself

Conform – to act or behave in the same way as the rest of a group

Consequences – the effects of our actions

Constipation – inability to have a bowel movement

Constriction – narrowing, making smaller

Consult – talk to others, ask for people's ideas and views

Consultant – a care worker who has qualifications and experience to specialise in particular conditions or diseases

Contract – a formal agreement between two or more people or organisations

Contribution – paying something towards

Controlled drugs – drugs that are limited by law

Cooperate – to work together

Culture – common values, beliefs and customs

DNA – (deoxyribonucleic acid) your body blueprint, found in the cells

Data Protection Act – law that is to do with information that is kept about clients

Debate – discussion; to talk about, to give views and opinions

Decision – a resolution, an outcome

Deficiency – less than is needed

Degenerative – where an organ, or body process slowly begins to break down or stop functioning

Dehydration – the body loses water and does not have enough to work properly

Demand – the amount of need for a service or treatment

Dementia – a condition that affects the working of the brain and blocks short-term memory

Dependable – trustworthy and reliable

Dependency – relying on

Dependent – needing help from others, not being able to do things for oneself

Depressant – a drug that slows down bodily function

Depression – feeling very unhappy or despondent

Diabetes insipidus – disease that stops the body properly using and regulating sugars

Diagnosis – identifying what the problem is

Diarrhoea – loose or fluid bowel movement

Dignity – self-respect

Diplomacy – being sensitive to the needs of others

Direct care role – a job with the responsibility for the care of patients or clients

Direct tax – money that is taken from our salary or wages before we receive it

Disadvantaged – unable to fulfill basic needs

Discrimination – to show bias or intolerance

Disloyalty – something that could cause you not to be trusted

Disoriented – not knowing which direction to take, or what is happening

Double vision – seeing two of everything

E. coli – type of bacterium

Early years services – care and education for children up to the age of eight years

Economic – anything that relates to money, for example, income, debt

Effluent – sewage and waste water

Egocentric – only able to see things from your own point of view

Emphysema – lung disease that destroys lung tissue and makes you short of breath

Empower – encourage people to be independent, not to have to rely on others

Environmental – to do with our surroundings

Epidemic – outbreak of disease in an area of people

Eradicate – remove completely

Ethnicity – our cultural background

Exception – something not like the norm

Expected – something you know is going to happen; planned

Fallopian tubes – the tubes that join ovaries to the uterus

Fallout – small radioactive particles that exist in the air after a nuclear explosion

Family ties – close links with family, loyalty

Flexibility – able to adapt; not having to keep to the same routine

Formal relationship – relationship, such as a working relationship, that has rules about how people should behave

Framework – structure or boundaries

Function – (verb) work; (noun) what something does

Fundamental – basic

Funding – providing money for services

Gender – denotes sex, male or female

Gender role – how men and women are expected to act in particular situations

Gene – part of a chromosome that controls a particular characteristic, eg. eye colour

Genetic disorder – disease or problem caused by our genes

Geriatric hospital – a hospital that specialises in caring for older people

Glaucoma – eye disease that may cause blindness

Goal – the purpose or target

Government – people that make political decisions about what should happen

Greenhouse effect – heating effect on the atmosphere

Gregarious – enjoy the company of others

Growth spurt – a rapid period of growth

Hallucination – seeing things that are not really there

Hazard – a danger

Health Action Zone (HAZ) – organisations in a particular area working together on identified projects to meet the needs of people living in the area

Health and social care – places or services that help to met our needs

Health authority – the organisation responsible for the health needs of people within an area

Health insurance policy – a way of saving towards the cost of having an operation or treatment with a private provider

Hereditary – characteristics passed from our parents

Heterosexual – someone who forms a sexual relationship with a member of the opposite sex

Holistic – to look at whole; to consider the whole person

Homosexual – someone who forms a sexual relationship with a member of the same sex

Hormone – chemical messenger that affects the way our bodies function

Hyperthermia – extremely high body temperature or fever (heat stroke)

Hypothermia – condition that develops when the body temperature falls

Identify – recognise

Immune system – body's system to protect against disease

Immunity – resistance to a disease

Impairment – condition that means we are not able-bodied

Income – the amount of money coming in to a person or to a home

Independent – able to do things without help

Indirect care role – helping to care for a patient or client by providing support

Indirect tax – a tax on items that we choose to buy

Individualised – designed for one person

Influence – an effect on a person

Informal relationship – casual or social relationship

Informed – having knowledge

Inhale – breathe in

Inherited – genetic information passed from parent to children

Inquisitive – curious, eager to learn

Intake – what is taken in

Intellect – the part of the brain that deals with thinking

Intense – strong

Interaction – being with other people and exchanging ideas

Intimate relationship – a very close and trusting relationship

Isolated – alone; cut off

Isolation – on its own

Issue – an important subject, requiring a decision

Joint working – organisations or people from different care sectors working together for the benefit of clients

Judgement – a decision about someone or something

Key worker – the main person who takes responsibility

Kilojoule – unit of energy

Laboratory – building or room equipped for scientific research or experiments

Leadership role – activity carried out by someone who leads or is in charge

Learning disability – a condition that prevents the brain working fully

Life expectancy – the average length of time that a person will live

Life experience – knowing about the wider world after being in school or college

Listeria – type of bacterium

Local authority – the organisation responsible for people within a local area

Located – placed or put

Lone parent – only one parent, a mother or father but not both, bringing up a child

Makaton – a type of sign language

Massage – using the hands to rub, knead and manipulate parts of the client's body

Mature – when a person's development is complete

Media – television, radio, newspapers, web sites, etc. that pass on information

Medication – tablets or other forms of drugs given to aid recovery

Menopause – the end of a woman's reproductive life

Minerals – chemicals, some of which are needed as nutrients in our diet

Minimum – least or lowest

Minister – a person from government who is put in charge of a department or a project

Miscarriage – natural abortion, loss of a fetus

Mobility – ability to move

Monitor – to keep a check on, or to keep an ongoing record of something

Morality – conforming to accepted standards of conduct in society

Mould – a type of fungus that grows in colonies or patches

Mutual support – two or more people sharing and helping each other

Mutual tolerance – where two or more people accept what the other is doing and have respect for their opinions

Named person – the person who has responsibility for liaising with other agencies

National insurance – money collected from our salary/wages to pay for public services

Nature – the qualities we are born with that make us what we are

Neighbourhood – area where a group of people lives

Nicotine – a stimulant chemical found in cigarettes

Non-statutory – not required by law

Non-verbal communication – not using speech, but using body language, such as smiling

Not-for-profit – not charging, or only charging enough money to cover costs

Nutrient – valuable part of our food

Nurture – how we are influenced when we are young by the environment around us, including other people

Obese – very overweight

Obesity – very overweight

Objective – something you set out to do

Observable – something that you can see

Observe – watch

Ophthalmic – relating to the eye

Oral hygienist – a person whose role is to attend to the hygiene of clients' teeth, gums and mouth

Organisation – a business or other concern, set up for a particular purpose

Organism – life form

Osteoporosis – condition related to bones caused by deficiency of calcium

Overcome – to get over a difficulty

Ozone layer – layer of gas that protects the planet from the sun's harmful rays

Pandemic – disease occurring worldwide

Particulate – microscopic particle

Participate – take part in

Partnership – relationship involving two or more individuals

Peak flow – the maximum rate at which you can expel (blow) air from your lungs

Peer group – people of the same age

Permanent – lasting for ever

Personal modesty – being reserved about exposing your body and in your sexual behaviour

Personality – the part of us that makes us an individual, who we are

Physical barrier – some material or object that prevents a person doing what they want to do, for example, a person in a wheelchair unable to get to a GP surgery because of steps

Physical measurement – height and weight or other measurement

Physiological measurement – blood pressure, peak flow or other body function measurement

Policy – a document that sets out the aims of the approach that is to be used

Population – the people who live in a place or area

Positive – concentrating on what is good

Potential – showing the possibility of achieving to the best of our ability

Poverty – being poor, not having much money

Power – having control, or a hold over someone

Practice – actually doing the job or work

Practitioner – someone who practises a profession

Premises – office or other building

Prescription – authorisation to obtain drugs given by a doctor

Pressure group – a group of people with similar ideas who want to influence political decision-making

Preventable – stoppable

Primary care group – GPs (general practitioners), community nurses and others who have joined together as a group to buy and provide services for their clients

Primary health care – care provided by a care worker such as a GP, usually the first person to help a client

Privacy – being private

Private – not by law, working to make a profit

Procedure – course of action that must be followed

Professional referral – being passed from one professional care worker to another for advice and/or treatment

Profit – making more money than the cost from providing services or goods

Promiscuous – having a lot of sexual partners

Promote – to put forward

Prone – likely to be affected by

Provide – to give or make available

Psychological – relating to the mind

Psychological barrier – fears or anxiety that prevent someone doing what they want

Puberty – the physical features of becoming sexually mature

Pulp cavity – centre of a tooth where the nerve is

Pulse – the wave passing along the arteries each time the heart beats

Quality – an aspect or characteristic

Quality time – time when a parent or carer concentrates on being with a child

Range – extent from highest to lowest

Reassurance – convincing a person effectively

Reduce – to cut down, to make smaller

Regulate – control

Relate – how you get on with people

Relationship – two or more people forming a special bond

Research – obtain information

Resources – those things that are needed, for example, materials, people or money

Respiratory – related to the process of breathing

Restricted – only seen by those who have permission, with a limited number of people

having access

Revitalise – to refresh

Rheumatism – painful muscles and joints

Rights – what is due to us

Role model – someone we observe or copy

Route – way of getting somewhere, for example, to a job; a pathway

Rural – a country area, not a city or built-up area

SI units – internationally agreed metric units of measurement

Sector – a part or division of something

Sedative – something that makes you sleepy

Sedentary – inactive; not getting very much exercise

Self-awareness – knowing ourselves, including our strengths and weaknesses

Self-concept – how we see or think about ourselves

Self-esteem – the value that you attach to yourself and your skills

Self-image – how a person sees himself or herself

Self-referral – taking yourself to see a health or social care or early years care worker

Semen – fluid that contains sperm

Service provider – organisation that supplies help in an organised way through people trained in health, social care or early years

Sex hormone – chemical messenger in the body that affects our sexual development and activities

Sexual partner – someone in an intimate physical relationship

Sibling – a brother or sister

Skill – having the ability or talent

Social isolation – separated from the community

Social learning theory – the theory that people learn ways of behaving by copying others

Specialised – trained person with specific skills to deal with particular situations

Spores – reproductive structures that grow into a new organism

Stability – things not changing, remaining the same

Stamina – ability to keep going

Standard – a level of quality

Statutory – by law

Stereotype – consider all people of a particular group as being the same

Stigma – something that does not present a good image of the person

Stimulate – to get the mind and body active

Stimulation – arousal or excitement

Stroke – the common name for effects of a broken blood vessel on the brain

Supplement – something extra, to add to

Supportive – giving help

Tar – thick, oily, poisonous substance

Target – something to aim for

Tax – collection of money by government

Temporary – for a short while

Third-party referral – someone else letting a health or social care or early years care worker know about a person's possible need

Tolerance – the body needs more of a drug to have the same effect

Toxic – poisonous

Toxin – harmful substance

Traumatic – deep shock, or upset

Trust – having confidence in a person

Unexpected – a surprise, not planned

Vaccination – using a substance to prevent disease

Vaccine – substance that is given to protect against disease

Values – worth or standards

Vermin – creatures that can carry disease, eg rats, cockroaches

Virus – group that are much smaller than bacteria and are likely to be harmful

Voluntary – usually working unpaid, giving services free

Volunteer – someone who works without charging for what they do

Vulnerable – at risk of harm

Wean – to introduce solid foods into a child's diet so that they are no longer dependent on milk

Working relationship – the bond you make when you work with someone

Index

Page numbers in green show where key words are given and explained.